Pregnancy & Birth

Everything you need to know

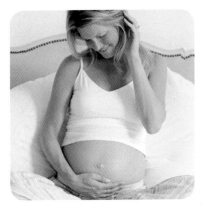

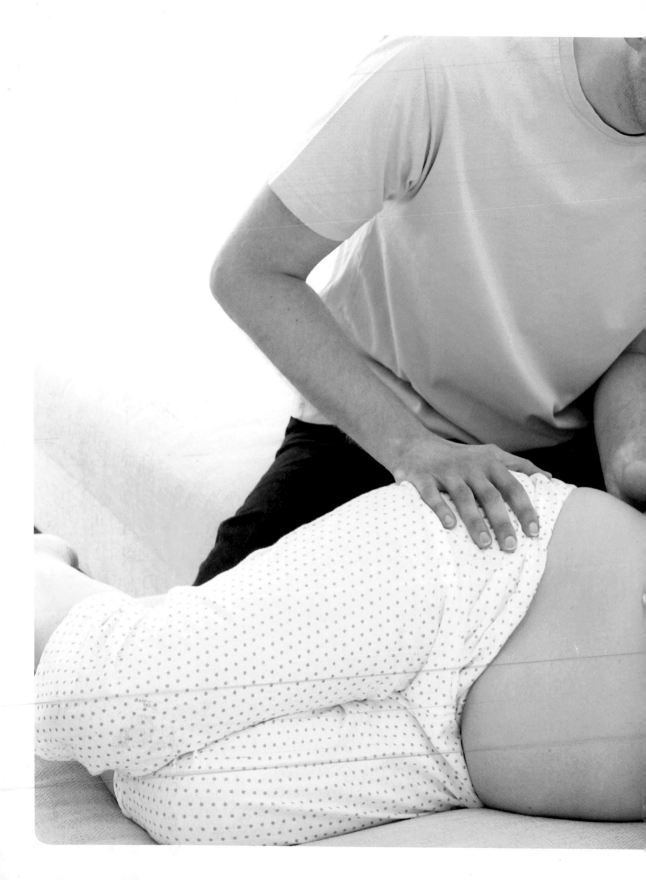

Pregnancy & Birth

Everything you need to know

Dr Mary Steen

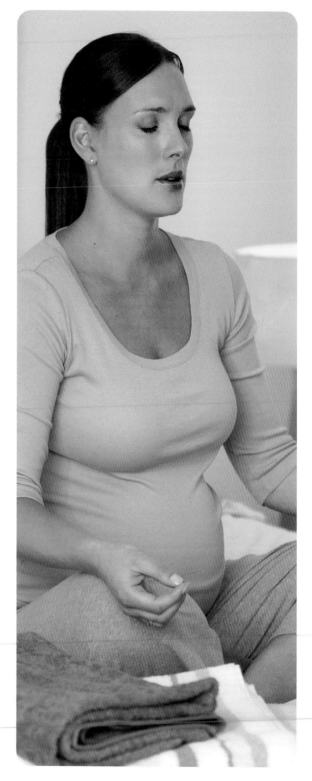

DK

London • New York • Munich • Melbourne • Delhi

Project editor Claire Tennant-Scull
Designer Carolyn Hewitson
Senior editor Helen Murray
Senior art editor Sara Kimmins
Design assistant Charlotte Johnson
Managing editor Penny Warren
Managing art editor Glenda Fisher
Production editor Maria Elia
Production controller Alice Sykes
Creative technical support Sonia Charbonnier
Art director Lisa Lanzarini
Category publisher Peggy Vance
Editorial consultant Karen Sullivan
Photographer Ruth Jenkinson
Photography art direction Peggy Sadler

Every effort has been made to ensure that the information contained in this book is complete and accurate. However, neither the publisher nor the author are engaged in rendering professional advice or services to the individual reader. The ideas, procedures, and suggestions contained in the book are not intended as a substitute for consultation with your healthcare provider. All matters regarding the health of you and your child require medical supervision. Neither the publisher nor the author accept any legal responsibility for any personal injury or other damage or loss arising from the use or misuse of the information and advice in this book.

First published in Great Britain in 2011 by Dorling Kindersley Limited, 80 Strand, London, WC2R 0RL Penguin Group (UK)

2 4 6 8 10 9 7 5 3 1

001 – 178166 – March 2011

A CIP catalogue of this book is available from the British Library

ISBN 978-1-4053-5818-7

Colour reproduction by Colourscan in Singapore
Printed and bound by Tien Wah Press in Singapore

Discover more at
www.dk.com

Contents

Your new baby

About the author

Dr Mary Steen is a mother of three children and has been practising as a midwife in the UK for over 20 years. Mary has undertaken several research studies with the aim of improving care and services for pregnant women, babies and their families. Her PhD focused specifically on the care and consequences of perineal trauma after childbirth and she invented a cooling device (Feme Pad) to alleviate pain caused by injury and stitches.

Mary presents at conferences nationally and internationally, and her work has been published in several health journals and books. She contributed to *Ask a Midwife* and *The Day-by-Day Pregnancy Book*, also published by Dorling Kindersley. Mary is the professional editor of the Royal College of Midwives midwifery magazine, and online papers, an editorial board member, and peer reviewer of midwifery journals, and a member of the Pampers Village Parenting Expert Panel.

Mary's work has received awards for clinical innovation, original research, and outstanding services to midwifery. In 2010, she was made Professor of Midwifery at the University of Chester.

Introduction

Being pregnant and giving birth are amazing experiences, which will change your life forever. You may be happy and excited about being pregnant, or, as recent research suggests, you may feel anxious, and rely on your family and friends to provide you with the information you need.

This is what prompted me to write this book; and this is a book with a difference – it's designed not only to help alleviate any concerns or anxiety you may have about pregnancy, birth, and parenthood, but to *show* you the very best ways to master each and every stage. I've been a midwife and a mum for many years, and I have included all the top tips that have made each of these experiences a success for the women I've had the pleasure of helping.

The book is divided into three sections: Pregnancy, Labour and Birth, and Your New Baby. The first section covers all aspects of your antenatal care, including what to expect during your pregnancy and the physical and emotional changes that you will experience. It will answer your questions on nutrition, exercise, your baby's development, and the preparations you'll need to make for your baby's arrival. Labour and Birth includes what to expect during labour and explains the birth process and the various options available to you, such as pain relief and where to give birth. Your New Baby explains the postnatal care and support you and your baby will receive, as well as babycare basics, for example, how to change a nappy, how to breastfeed, and advice on establishing sleep patterns.

Remember that women have been giving birth for thousands and thousands of years, and we'll continue to do so. Pregnancy and birth are normal, healthy life events. Have confidence in your own ability to give birth and become a parent, and don't be afraid to ask for help and advice.

Today, I am as enthusiastic about being a midwife as I was when I first registered over 20 years ago. I am delighted to be able to pass on the knowledge I have accrued over the years. Enjoy, and I wish you all the best.

Dr Mary Steen
Professor of Midwifery, University of Chester, UK

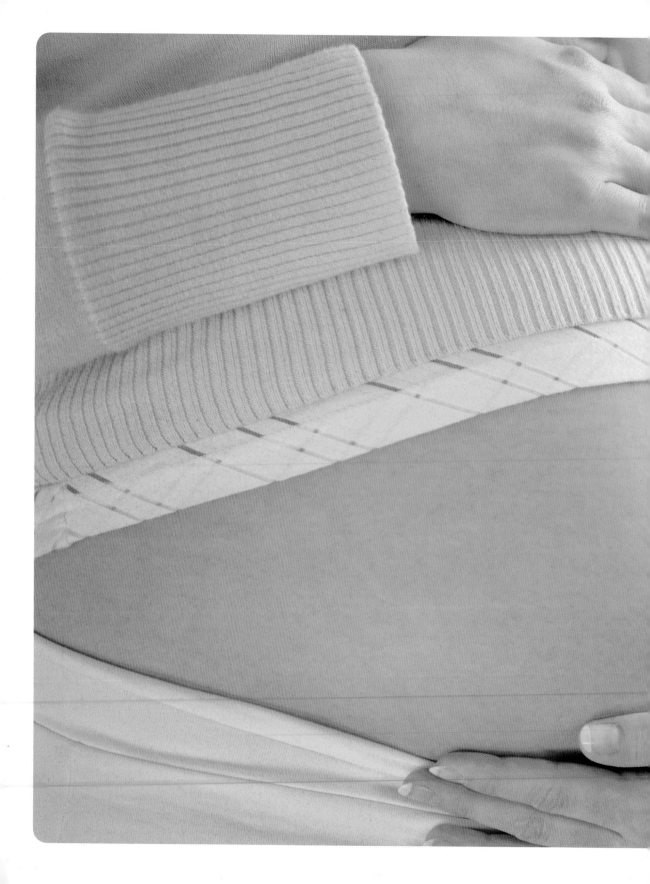

Pregnancy

YOUR PREGNANCY

Becoming pregnant is one of the most amazing, life-changing events for any couple. It is completely normal to experience some anxiety and concern, but rest assured that you will soon come to terms with your new status, and begin to enjoy your role as an expectant parent.

NOW YOU'RE PREGNANT

Pregnancy is a time of change for all women, whether a baby is part of your long-term plans, or an unexpected surprise. As hormones begin to surge through your body, and you adapt to the demands of your growing baby, you'll be faced with a number of decisions, and an exciting list of arrangements to make as you prepare for your new baby. You'll need to think through the type of antenatal care you want, and how and where you'd like your baby to be born. You'll need to consider the best way to juggle work and impending motherhood, and fit in the all-essential antenatal appointments and tests that will help to make sure that both you and your baby stay healthy and well.

LOOK AFTER YOURSELF

You'll need to take good care of yourself, eating and drinking well, getting plenty of fresh air, light exercise, and restful sleep, and relaxing whenever you can, to give your baby the best possible start in life. You may find that you experience a host of symptoms, and wonder if they're normal – or if they'll ever end! You may feel up, down, and all over the place emotionally, too. Over the coming pages, we'll look at the various ways to find a healthy balance in your life, get the support you need, and answer those niggling questions that sit firmly on the edges of your mind.

YOUR BABY

Best of all, we'll show you exactly how your baby will develop over the coming months and look at the changes that will occur to your body as your pregnancy moves forward. We'll also get you started with preparations for that all-important day when you welcome your baby home.

THE FIRST TRIMESTER

Pregnancy is roughly divided into three stages, known as "trimesters". The first trimester, which runs from conception until 12 weeks, can be the most trying for some women. Not only is it common to experience symptoms such as morning sickness, constipation, headaches, and breast tenderness, but you may feel a little out of sorts emotionally – experiencing elation one moment, and inexplicable anxiety or tearfulness the next. Your baby will grow and develop at a dramatic rate, and by just 10–12 weeks, he'll have all of his body parts in place and your placenta will be fully developed and able to sustain him for the duration of your pregnancy.

The first trimester also marks a series of appointments, tests, and procedures that forms the foundation of your antenatal care, and you'll be given plenty of guidance, support, and information to help you make informed decisions and choices throughout your pregnancy, and the birth itself. These are exciting weeks, and you'll be surrounded by professionals who will make sure that your pregnancy progresses as it should.

THE SECOND TRIMESTER

This runs between weeks 13 and 27, and many women report feeling energetic and balanced during this period. Your body will have adapted to the hormonal changes, and

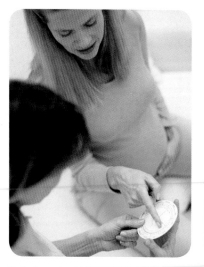

Help is on hand Make the most of the wide range of support available to you and don't be afraid to ask questions at any stage.

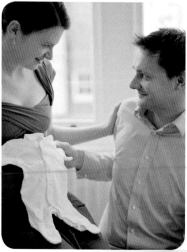

Getting ready Use the months of your pregnancy to get everything in place, ready for the arrival of your baby.

experience fewer unpleasant symptoms, and you may find that your skin and hair glow with good health. It's more than likely that your bump will "show" during this period, and you will also feel your baby's first movements. You may experience the first "practice" contractions, known as Braxton Hicks'.

THE THIRD TRIMESTER

From 28 weeks, you will have entered your third and final trimester of pregnancy, when the growing weight of your baby – and the demands placed on your body – can leave you feeling tired and uncomfortable. Your body will be gearing up for the birth, and you'll also begin to make the final preparations for childbirth and getting everything in place to welcome your new baby home. For some women, the reality of having a baby in the house only hits now.

GETTING THE SUPPORT YOU NEED

No two pregnancies are ever the same, and you may find that you have a host of niggling questions and concerns as the weeks progress. The good news is that you will have a built-in "circle of care" – midwives, doctors, and nurses who will provide you with plenty of opportunities to ask questions and get the support you need. There is a great deal of research to suggest that women who are well informed go on to have the most positive pregnancies and easiest labours, so don't hesitate to ask for help if you need it.

A LITTLE ORGANIZATION

We'll look at everything you need to know to negotiate your pregnancy with ease, and make the right choices for you and your baby. By the time you go into labour, you'll have everything in place to welcome your baby home. And, by getting things organized a little at a time, you'll be calm, relaxed, and well prepared for the changes to come.

Pregnancy is a time of great joy and anticipation. By staying positive, getting to grips with the basics, and taking steps to make sure that everything progresses the way you want it to, you can settle back to enjoy the coming months, and enter the next phase of your life with confidence.

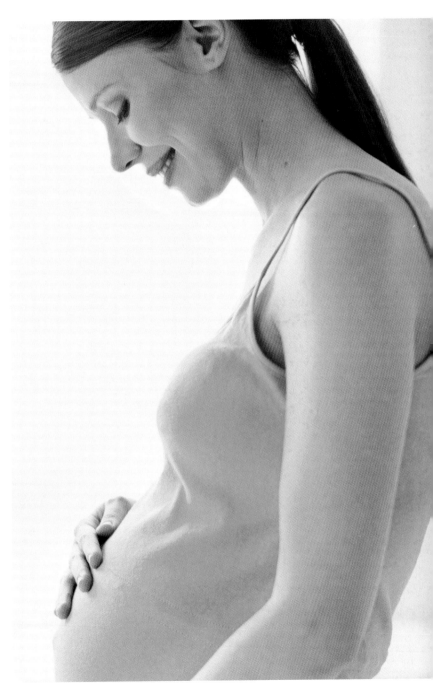

Take care of yourself It is important to look after yourself throughout your pregnancy – eat well, take light exercise, and focus on being as healthy as possible. And make time to savour the experience – once your baby is here, you may get little time to yourself.

Now you are pregnant

Whether you've been trying for a baby for some time, or you find yourself unexpectedly pregnant, the amazing news that you are expecting a baby heralds a new and exciting phase of your life.

A positive test

It's perfectly normal to experience many different emotions as you get to grips with your new role as an expectant parent.

Get support Pregnancy is an exciting and challenging time for many women and men, and it's important that you get some support to deal with the changes that you will be experiencing both physically and emotionally. Telling a few family members or close friends will give you an opportunity to share any concerns and get some answers to questions that are sure to crop up over the next few weeks.

Join in You may wish to sign up to a website that will give you regular pregnancy updates – keeping you posted on what's happening to your body, and how your baby will be growing and developing. Websites often have communities of parents who are keen to discuss the intricacies of pregnancy and new parenthood, and you may find this an invaluable source of reassurance and information.

Enjoy your pregnancy It may seem hard to believe, but the next nine months will fly by and it won't be long before you have your new baby in your arms.

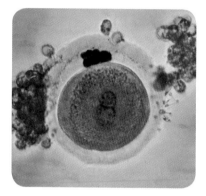

A new life Just 24 hours after conception, your egg and your partner's sperm will be on their way to creating the embryo that will become your baby. Your hormone levels have already begun to change, and you may experience nausea and breast tenderness.

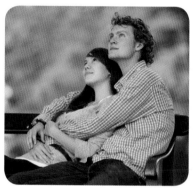

Shared excitement Although you may be bursting to tell everyone, it may be wise to wait a little while longer. For a variety of reasons, some pregnancies do not progress. Waiting until the 12th week will allow you to share your news with confidence.

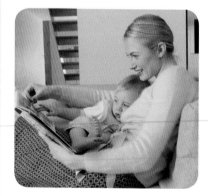

Choose the right time Any other children you have will be excited about the prospect of a little brother or sister, but it's worth holding off telling them until later in your pregnancy. While it's good to prepare them, it's hard for children to understand the wait.

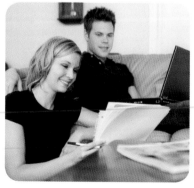

Big decisions Some major decisions must be made over the coming months, and it's important that you talk things through with your partner. You may both be feeling a little overwhelmed, but expressing your feelings will strengthen your relationship.

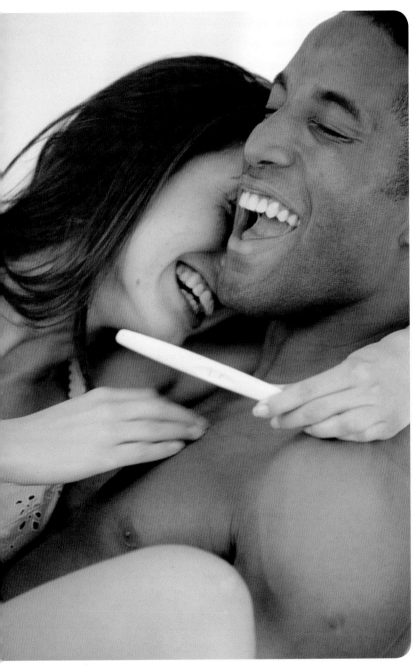

Life-changing news Don't be surprised if you swing between feelings of elation and anxiety. Becoming pregnant is a miraculous event and a momentous occasion, but it does mark the beginning of a whole new stage of your life. This may take some getting used to, so give yourself and your partner plenty of time to adjust to the news.

What happens now?

Before you head straight to the baby department of your local store, there are some practical things you can do to get your pregnancy off to a flying start.

Folic acid If you are not already doing so, you should begin taking this supplement, which is essential for your baby's healthy development. Folic acid is a B vitamin (B_9) found mostly in leafy green vegetables such as kale and spinach, orange juice, and enriched grains. Numerous studies have shown that women who get 400mcg per day, prior to conception and during early pregnancy, reduce the risk of neural tube birth defects by up to 70 per cent.

Be safe If your pregnancy was planned, the chances are that alcohol and smoking have been off the menu for some time. If you haven't already given up, now is the time to do so. It's also time to make sure that your diet is healthy and balanced, with plenty of fresh, whole foods to supply your baby with the nutrients she needs to grow and develop.

Make it official Let your doctor or midwife know that you are expecting, and set up an appointment to "book in" (see pp.18–19) for your first antenatal appointment. You could also look for antenatal classes, as good ones fill up fast.

Begin a pregnancy diary Use this to note how you are feeling and what symptoms you are experiencing. Ask your partner or a friend to take a photo every month to keep a record of your changing body.

Your antenatal care

You will soon begin to receive regular antenatal care designed to monitor the health of both you and your baby. There are several different care options available, but the important thing is to get the type of care that you want.

What to expect

Expect these routine appointments with your midwife or doctor:

★ 6–8 weeks – first contact.

★ 10–12 weeks – "booking appointment" (see pp.18–19).

★ Then at: 16 weeks, 25 weeks, 28 weeks, 31 weeks, 34 weeks, 36 weeks, 38 weeks, 40 weeks, and 41 weeks (if you are overdue).

Blood tests:

★ 10 weeks (see pp.19 & 56).

Routine scans: (see pp.54–55).

★ 10–14 weeks to confirm dates and detect twins.

★ 18–20 weeks to check your baby's development and the placenta's position.

★ You may have more if your pregnancy is high risk (see pp.58–59).

Screening tests:

★ 11–16 weeks – a "triple" or "quadruple" blood test to check for Spina Bifida, Down's syndrome, and Edward's syndrome.

★ If your pregnancy is considered to carry some risk factors (see pp.58–59), you may have the combination of a nuchal translucency (NT) scan (see p.56) and blood tests.

Diagnostic tests:

★ If screening tests suggest a high risk of chromosomal abnormalities, you may be offered further tests to establish whether or not an abnormality is present (see p.56).

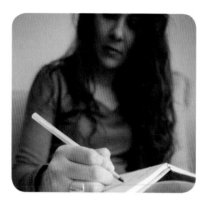

Questions or concerns Before your first antenatal contact, write a list of questions. Developing a trusting relationship with your midwife or doctor will go a long way towards helping you to have greater confidence throughout your pregnancy.

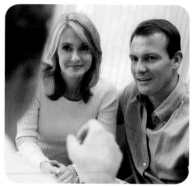

Attending appointments You will have regular antenatal appointments over the coming months, and you are legally allowed time off work to go to them. You may wish to include your partner sometimes to give him an opportunity to ask questions, too.

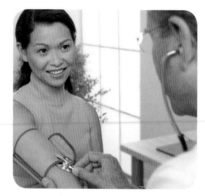

Test and scans You will have regular tests as well as one or more scans (see pp.54–55), even if you are in glowing good health. The purpose of these is to make sure that both you and your baby are healthy and well, and that your pregnancy is progressing as it should.

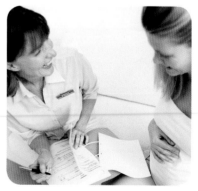

Midwives You may be introduced to a midwife – or a team of midwives – who will undertake the majority of your antenatal care. Some women hire an independent midwife to make sure that they have continuity of care. Ask what's available in your area.

Estimated date of delivery

Until you have a dating scan, (see pp.54–55), you can find your estimated date of delivery (EDD) by using this chart. Find the date of the first day of your last menstrual period (LMP) shown here in bold. The date shown in lighter type underneath this will tell you when your baby is expected.

January	1	2	3	4	5	6	7	8	9	10	11	12	13	14	15	16	17	18	19	20	21	22	23	24	25	26	27	28	29	30	31
Oct/Nov	8	9	10	11	12	13	14	15	16	17	18	19	20	21	22	23	24	25	26	27	28	29	30	31	1	2	3	4	5	6	7
February	1	2	3	4	5	6	7	8	9	10	11	12	13	14	15	16	17	18	19	20	21	22	23	24	25	26	27	28			
Nov/Dec	8	9	10	11	12	13	14	15	16	17	18	19	20	21	22	23	24	25	26	27	28	29	30	1	2	3	4	5			
March	1	2	3	4	5	6	7	8	9	10	11	12	13	14	15	16	17	18	19	20	21	22	23	24	25	26	27	28	29	30	31
Dec/Jan	6	7	8	9	10	11	12	13	14	15	16	17	18	19	20	21	22	23	24	25	26	27	28	29	30	31	1	2	3	4	5
April	1	2	3	4	5	6	7	8	9	10	11	12	13	14	15	16	17	18	19	20	21	22	23	24	25	26	27	28	29	30	
Jan/Feb	6	7	8	9	10	11	12	13	14	15	16	17	18	19	20	21	22	23	24	25	26	27	28	29	30	31	1	2	3	4	
May	1	2	3	4	5	6	7	8	9	10	11	12	13	14	15	16	17	18	19	20	21	22	23	24	25	26	27	28	29	30	31
Feb/Mar	5	6	7	8	9	10	11	12	13	14	15	16	17	18	19	20	21	22	23	24	25	26	27	28	1	2	3	4	5	6	7
June	1	2	3	4	5	6	7	8	9	10	11	12	13	14	15	16	17	18	19	20	21	22	23	24	25	26	27	28	29	30	
Mar/Apr	8	9	10	11	12	13	14	15	16	17	18	19	20	21	22	23	24	25	26	27	28	29	30	31	1	2	3	4	5	6	
July	1	2	3	4	5	6	7	8	9	10	11	12	13	14	15	16	17	18	19	20	21	22	23	24	25	26	27	28	29	30	31
Apr/May	7	8	9	10	11	12	13	14	15	16	17	18	19	20	21	22	23	24	25	26	27	28	29	30	1	2	3	4	5	6	7
August	1	2	3	4	5	6	7	8	9	10	11	12	13	14	15	16	17	18	19	20	21	22	23	24	25	26	27	28	29	30	31
May/June	8	9	10	11	12	13	14	15	16	17	18	19	20	21	22	23	24	25	26	27	28	29	30	31	1	2	3	4	5	6	7
September	1	2	3	4	5	6	7	8	9	10	11	12	13	14	15	16	17	18	19	20	21	22	23	24	25	26	27	28	29	30	
June/July	8	9	10	11	12	13	14	15	16	17	18	19	20	21	22	23	24	25	26	27	28	29	30	1	2	3	4	5	6	7	
October	1	2	3	4	5	6	7	8	9	10	11	12	13	14	15	16	17	18	19	20	21	22	23	24	25	26	27	28	29	30	31
July/Aug	8	9	10	11	12	13	14	15	16	17	18	19	20	21	22	23	24	25	26	27	28	29	30	31	1	2	3	4	5	6	7
November	1	2	3	4	5	6	7	8	9	10	11	12	13	14	15	16	17	18	19	20	21	22	23	24	25	26	27	28	29	30	
Aug/Sept	8	9	10	11	12	13	14	15	16	17	18	19	20	21	22	23	24	25	26	27	28	29	30	31	1	2	3	4	5	6	
December	1	2	3	4	5	6	7	8	9	10	11	12	13	14	15	16	17	18	19	20	21	22	23	24	25	26	27	28	29	30	31
Sept/Oct	7	8	9	10	11	12	13	14	15	16	17	18	19	20	21	22	23	24	25	26	27	28	29	30	1	2	3	4	5	6	7

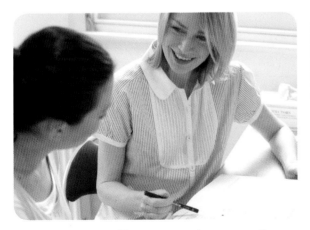

Routine appointments You can expect to have seven to 10 appointments, as well as scans and tests. If your pregnancy is high risk (see pp.58–59), you may be referred to an obstetrician.

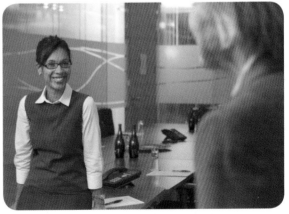

Telling your boss Although you may wish to keep your pregnancy a secret for now, you will need to inform your employer, in order to be able to take time off work for antenatal appointments.

Antenatal care options

In the UK, most women receive their antenatal care from a community midwife, either in their own home, at a health centre, or GP's surgery.

Questions to ask your midwife

Don't be embarrassed about asking questions; it is your midwife's job to make sure that you are happy and informed throughout your pregnancy. You may wish to ask:

★ Where can I have my baby?

★ Can I have a home or water birth?

★ Can I use natural remedies and therapies, and what is the hospital or maternity unit policy for the use of these?

★ What analgesics and other medications are safe during pregnancy?

★ Are my symptoms normal?

★ I've had some spotting. Will my baby be all right?

★ What do the results of my tests and screens mean?

★ Who should I call if I am worried or something goes wrong?

★ Who should I call when I go into labour?

★ Will I see the same midwife at every appointment?

★ Will I have the same midwife for my entire labour?

★ Can I say no to interventions during labour, and if so, which?

★ Can I have an elective Caesarean?

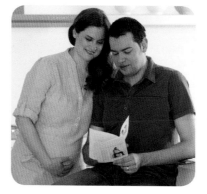

Research your options Early in your pregnancy, it's a good idea to think about how and where you will give birth.

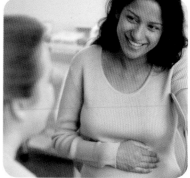

Your midwife She will be happy to answer any questions that you may have, and will be able to help you to deal with any concerns.

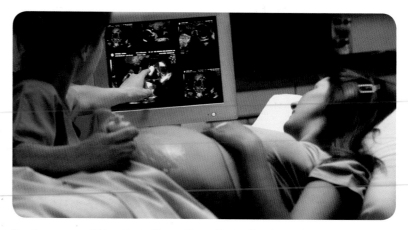

Routine scans and blood tests These will usually take place in your local hospital. In some cases, you can choose the hospital you attend, and where you'll eventually give birth. It's worth asking what's available, and talk to other mums, too, to hear about their experiences.

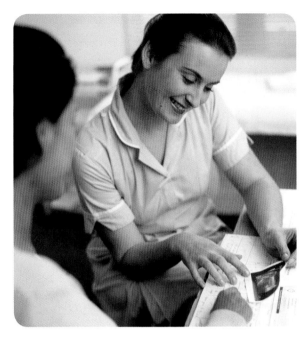

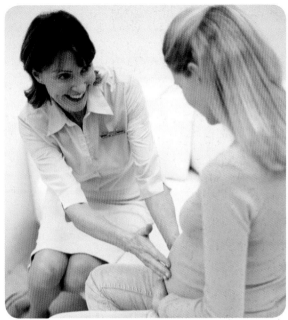

Results These will be discussed with you at every stage of your pregnancy, but ask if you're unsure about something. If the results aren't as expected, you may be referred to an obstetrician, who can keep an eye on a higher-risk pregnancy (see pp.58–59).

Home appointments Many women choose to have their antenatal appointments at home – sometimes with a view to having a home birth. This option may be available to you; if it's not, you might hire an independent midwife who will be able to be more flexible.

Natural pregnancy

Many women choose to eat fresh, organic foods that are free from pesticides and other chemicals, and forego any medication that could harm their baby. As a result, there is a burgeoning industry of products and services designed for women who want a natural pregnancy and birth.

Natural antenatal care options
Alongside the usual care provided by your midwife or doctor, you may wish to see a natural-health practitioner, such as a homoeopath, a herbalist, an acupuncturist, a reflexologist or an aromatherapist. Not only can they help to make sure that you remain healthy throughout your pregnancy, but a good practitioner can address many of the uncomfortable symptoms you may be experiencing.

Safe care Many therapies are perfectly safe in pregnancy, but you must make sure that you find an experienced, registered practitioner who is aware of any regular health problems that you may have. It's equally important to keep your usual antenatal care provider in the loop; they will need to know of any remedies that you are taking, and what treatments you are receiving. A good practitioner can offer support and advice throughout your pregnancy and may even be able to provide you with some tools and techniques to help you cope with labour.

A natural birth If you have your heart set on a natural birth, you can also enlist the services of an independent midwife who promotes this approach, or arrange to have your baby at a birth centre. Most midwives are very sensitive to the fact that many women wish to keep things as natural as possible, throughout the antenatal period and beyond, and will be happy to support your decisions. It is important to remember, however, that any complications or problems that arise during pregnancy – and throughout labour – may need medical interventions. Try to remain flexible, and remember that your ultimate goal is to deliver a healthy baby, by whatever means necessary.

Your booking appointment

After your "first contact" appointment, your next proper meeting with your midwife is known as the "booking" appointment. You can expect to talk through your medical history and the choices you have for your antenatal care and the birth, and you will also have some routine tests to check that all is well.

Being prepared

★ **It's worth checking** with your own parents to establish what childhood diseases or immunizations you have had.

★ **Ask your partner** his blood type before your visit; if you are Rhesus-negative and he is Rhesus-positive you could build up antibodies against your baby. There is an injection that you can have to prevent this (see p.57).

★ **Make a note** of the first day of your last period, which will allow your midwife to calculate your due date.

★ **Be prepared** to be honest; you need to tell your midwife if you smoke, and how much alcohol you drink. Both of these can affect your baby's health.

KEY FACT
Your midwife will not yet offer an internal examination or even feel your abdomen; this type of "palpation" does not normally take place until after about 24 weeks.

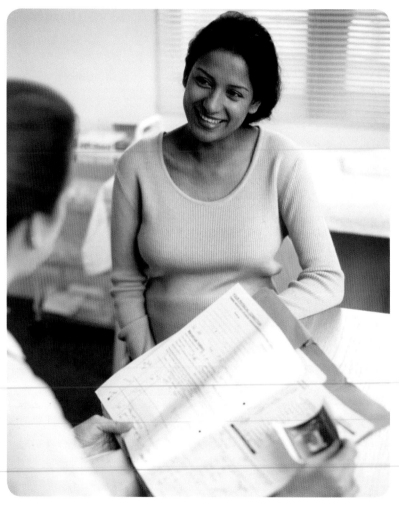

Your care Your booking appointment will take place at around 10 to 12 weeks. In some areas, this is done at home by a community midwife; in others, you'll be asked to visit the hospital or your GP's surgery. You'll need to have a clear idea of your medical history.

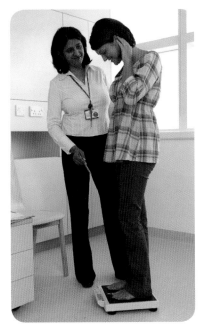

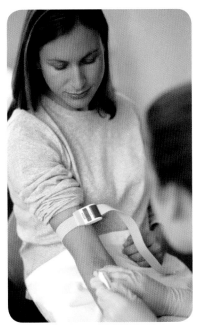

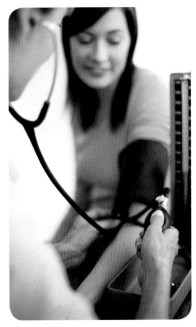

Weight You will be weighed during your booking appointment, to work out your BMI (body mass index). This can help to prevent certain risk factors in women with a low or high BMI, allowing your midwife to plan your care to suit you and your body.

Blood tests These will be undertaken or arranged at your first appointment, in order to establish your general level of health and even your baby's (see below). Some of the tests are optional, and you can talk to your GP or midwife about your choices.

Blood pressure This will be taken at every antenatal appointment, to check that it stays within safe parameters. Measurements can fluctuate throughout pregnancy but your midwife will be looking at general trends and watching for any changes.

What to expect

Your first contact and booking appointments allow your midwife to get a clear idea of your health, medical history, and the type of antenatal care and birth you want. She'll explain the reasons for the tests and procedures that will be necessary. You can expect to talk about:

★ Your lifestyle habits: smoking, drinking, diet, and exercise.
★ Your health: are you overweight? Taking any medication? Suffering from any chronic or short-term problems?
★ Your medical history: including your family's medical history. Are there any genetic conditions that run in your family? Did your mum experience any complications during her pregnancy?
★ Your obstetric health: including previous miscarriages, abortions, and births. This may affect the options you

have for the birth, and define the type of care that may be required.
★ Your ethnic background: some health conditions, such as sickle-cell disease or thalassaemia, are more common among certain ethnic groups.
★ Screening tests (see pp.56–57): you do not have to have these tests if you do not want to.
★ Your sexual partners: this is to explore the possibility that you could be carrying a sexually transmitted disease.
★ Your birth choices: such as where and

how you want to have your baby.
★ How you intend to feed your baby: providing information about breastfeeding early on has been proved to encourage its success.
★ Your weight and your blood pressure (see above).
★ You'll also have a urine test, (see above and pp.56–57) and blood tests will be undertaken or arranged (see pp.56–57). Your midwife will take notes throughout the process, and a picture of your and your baby's overall health will emerge.

Staying healthy

Taking steps to achieve optimum health and wellbeing in your pregnancy will not only make it a positive experience, but you'll have fewer symptoms, an easier labour, and you'll look after the health of your baby, too.

Taking a balanced approach

Remember that what your baby needs most is a healthy, happy, relaxed mum. So enjoy your pregnancy!

Being sensible Most women are happy to adapt their lifestyles to ensure the health of their growing babies, but it's important not to go overboard. Strict diets or exercise routines can deplete your energy and leave you tired and frustrated. The very best advice is to enjoy the wonderful experience of being pregnant, and embrace the positive responsibility of providing your baby with the best possible conditions for his growth and development.

A healthy pregnancy In a nutshell, this means getting lots of sleep, plenty of fluids, fresh air and a little sunshine, some good, regular exercise, and a healthy diet. You'll also need to take time for your close relationships, which will become more important than ever when your new baby arrives. You may be tired and a little anxious from time to time, but keeping yourself in good health and trying to avoid placing too many demands on yourself, can make the whole process that much easier.

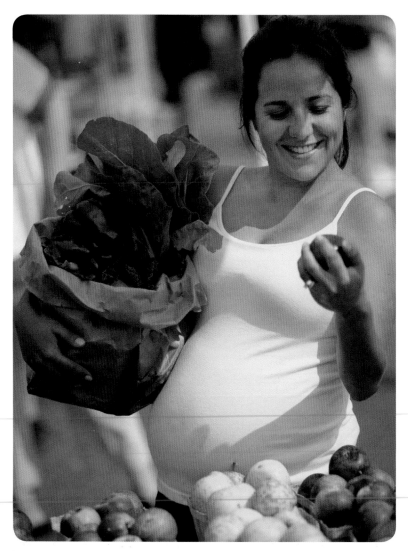

Better choices A healthy diet with plenty of fresh fruit and vegetables is essential. Food that is rich in nutrients will help to make sure that your baby gets everything he needs.

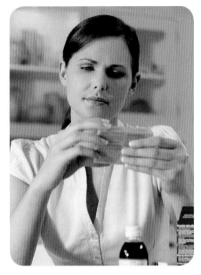

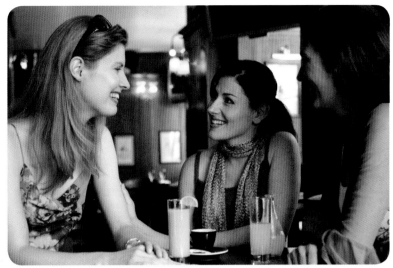

Medication Check with your doctor or midwife if you are taking regular medication; some should not be taken in pregnancy, and your prescription may need to be adjusted.

Lifestyle changes Now that you are pregnant, you will need to make a few adjustments. The effect of alcohol on your developing baby is not entirely clear, but the best advice is to give it up altogether. Smoking has been proven to cause health problems in unborn babies, so get some help to stop, if you haven't done so already.

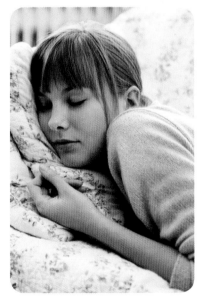

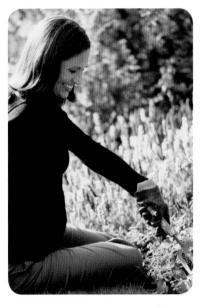

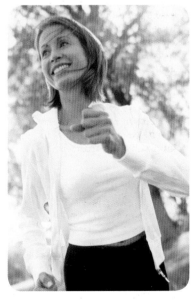

Getting plenty of restful sleep This will help you to cope with the many physical and emotional demands that pregnancy will make of you. Proper rest will also help you to maintain a positive attitude.

Taking care It's great to continue doing the hobbies you enjoy, getting regular, gentle exercise and lots of fresh air. But you may wish to check with your midwife to be sure that they are not hazardous in any way.

Exercise Now is not the time to begin a rigorous get-fit routine. However, regular exercise is important for a healthy pregnancy, so continue with your usual activities, with a few exceptions (see p.26).

Eating for two

A healthy diet not only keeps you alert and bursting with energy, but it reduces the risk of pregnancy complications and helps to make sure that your baby gets all of the nutrients she needs for optimum growth and development.

Foods to avoid during pregnancy

Take care to avoid these foods as they may present a variety of hazards:

★ Liver and cod liver oil, which can provide too much of the animal form of vitamin A, which has been found to be linked to birth defects.

★ Meat pâtés, which can be contaminated with food-borne illnesses.

★ Unpasteurized soft or blue cheese, such as camembert, goat's cheese, brie, and Stilton, which can contain listeria.

★ Raw or partially cooked eggs, including mayonnaise which can contain salmonella.

★ Raw or undercooked meat, fish and poultry, which can contain salmonella or *Toxoplasma gondii,* which can cause toxoplasmosis.

★ Ready-to-eat-salads in bags, which carry a risk of listeria.

★ Too much oily fish, which can contain pollutants such as dioxins, mercury, and chemicals such as PCBs (polychlorinated biphenyls). To be safe, limt yourself to two servings a week.

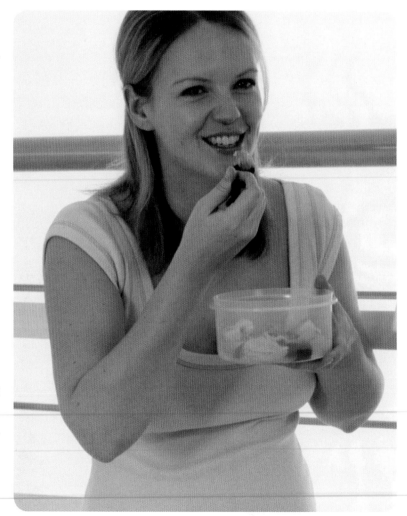

Refuelling Eating regularly is very important during pregnancy. You'll probably be hungrier than usual, and feel dizzy and out of sorts if your blood-sugar levels drop too low. Small, nutritious snacks, eaten throughout the day, and a good breakfast first thing in the morning, will give you the energy you need, and help to ease nausea.

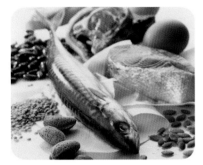

Protein Vital for the development of every new cell in your baby's body, protein is found in pulses, whole grains, nuts, soya, dairy produce, eggs, meats, poultry, and fish.

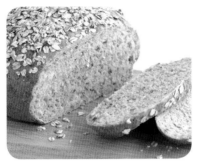

Whole grains These will give you a sustained source of energy and help keep your blood-sugar levels stable. They are also a fantastic source of fibre.

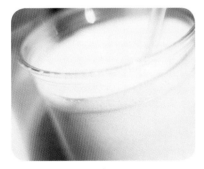

Calcium This is essential for your baby's bones and teeth. You'll find it in dairy products, soya, leafy green vegetables, and some fish, such as tinned salmon.

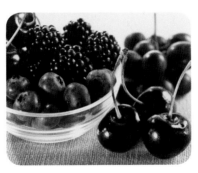

Fresh fruit As well as being packed with vitamins and minerals, these also provide fibre to keep your bowel movements regular and help you to absorb nutrients during digestion.

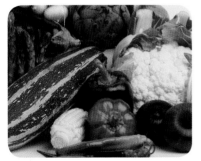

Brightly coloured and dark-green vegetables These are packed with vitamins and minerals that will help to maintain the health of both you and your baby. Aim for at least five servings a day.

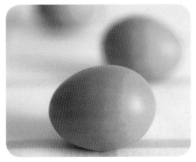

Eggs An excellent source of good-quality protein, eggs also contain some iron, which is particularly important during pregnancy. Take care to make sure that they are properly cooked though (see opposite).

Superfoods for pregnancy

The following foods should form the basis of your healthy pregnancy diet:

★ Whole grains, such as wholemeal bread and pasta, brown rice, pulses, and grains (such as barley, oats, and quinoa), to provide a sustained source of energy, plenty of fibre, and essential B vitamins.

★ Good-quality protein plays an extremely important part in your pregnancy and the development of your baby. Aim to consume about 70g (2½ oz) per day, particularly in the second and third trimesters, when your baby is growing quickly.

★ Healthy fats Fats are an important part of your diet, providing energy and vital nutrients. Aim to get plenty of essential fatty acids (EFAs), which are necessary for your baby's development, particularly her nervous system, brain, and vision. Good sources include well-cooked eggs, flaxseeds (and their oil), nuts, seeds, and oily fish (such as salmon and mackerel). Avoid trans fats (synthetically produced fats), and limit the saturated fats you eat.

★ Lots of fibre, to make sure that nutrients are efficiently absorbed, and your bowel movements are regular. Whole grains, fresh fruit, and vegetables should give you plenty.

KEY FACT
Vitamin D is extremely important in pregnancy yet many women are deficient. Getting plenty of sunshine and taking 10mcg per day can help to make sure you get enough.

Your pregnancy diet

Once you include healthy foods in your diet, you'll find that it's easy to eat well, and you'll immediately reap the benefits. Choose fresh, whole foods when you can, and avoid processed foods that will fill you with empty calories.

Folic acid and other supplements

Ask your doctor or midwife about what you may need.

Folic acid This is essential for the healthy development of your baby's nervous system. A healthy diet should contain good levels of this key nutrient, but it is recommended that all pregnant women take a supplement of 400mcg per day.

Iron Your need for iron is much higher than usual during pregnancy, so iron supplements may be required to keep your haemoglobin levels high.

Multi-vitamin and mineral tablets Take ones that are for use in pregnancy, especially if your diet is not quite as good as it should be.

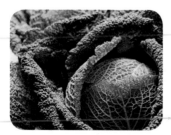

Leafy green vegetables These are a great source of essential fibre, vitamins, and folic acid.

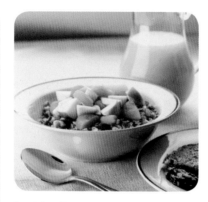

Breakfast Even if you aren't usually a big fan of breakfast, you will need to give your body a good dose of nutrients in the morning. Choose foods such as whole grain toast, fresh fruit, and perhaps some cereal or yogurt, to give you sustained energy.

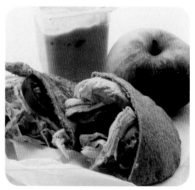

A healthy lunch Across the day you'll need a range of nutrients, so include plenty of whole grains, fruit, and vegetables, as well as a little protein. Take time to sit down for lunch. If you tend to eat at your desk, pack a lunch and take it with you to work.

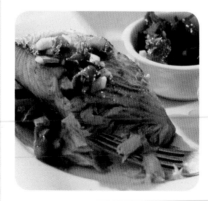

Evening meal A nutritious meal will help you to sleep, and can even help to prevent morning sickness by keeping your blood-sugar levels stable throughout the night. A little of each food group, with lots of fresh vegetables and whole grains is ideal.

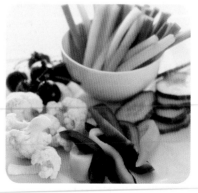

Eat little and often Not only does your blood sugar have a tendency to dip and soar during pregnancy, leaving you feeling tired and lethargic, but your body needs regular refuelling to keep up with the demands placed on it. Choose healthy snacks.

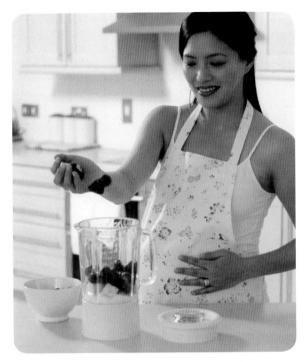

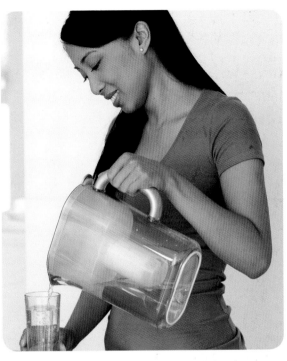

Smoothies If you are struggling to eat enough fruit, why not whizz up a smoothie, throwing in a few fresh vegetables such as carrots and spinach as well. If you add some yogurt or a little milk, you'll get some essential calcium, too. Smoothies are a great nutritious snack, or a good breakfast if you are on the run.

Drink plenty of fresh water This will not only help to keep symptoms such as nausea, headaches, and oedema (swelling) at bay, but it will keep you hydrated, improving your energy levels. Your fluid requirements increase dramatically during pregnancy, so aim to drink at least eight glasses per day.

Essential vitamins and minerals

A healthy, balanced diet should really provide you with all the vitamins and minerals you need during pregnancy. A whole spectrum of nutrients is essential; however, there are some key ones that are particularly important for your health and that of your developing baby.

Vitamin C This not only helps your body to fight infection and encourages the absorption of iron, but it is essential for the growth of a strong placenta that will sustain your baby throughout your pregnancy. Fresh fruit (especially raw) and vegetables will provide you with plenty.

Iron Although required throughout your pregnancy, iron becomes extremely important in the second and third trimesters, when you not only need it to make blood for you and your baby, but also to lay down stores in his body, which he will draw on for the first six months of life. Iron-rich foods help to prevent anaemia, which can be debilitating and potentially dangerous. Choose both plant and animal sources, as the latter are more easily absorbed. You'll find iron in lean red meats, leafy green vegetables, fish, dried fruits, beets, molasses, whole-grain bread, the dark skin of poultry, and iron-fortified cereals.

Calcium This is necessary for your baby's bones and teeth – and yours! It is also essential for the efficient functioning of your baby's heart, nerves, and muscles, and will help him to establish a normal heart rhythm and to aid blood-clotting. If you don't extract enough calcium from your diet when you are pregnant, your baby will have to get what he needs from your bones, which can cause problems, such as osteoporosis (brittle bones), for you later on.

Keeping fit

Exercise has a host of benefits during pregnancy – for both you and your baby. It is important to choose the type of exercise that you do carefully, but gentle, regular exercise will get your endorphins flowing and you'll feel fantastic.

Staying safe

★ **Don't exercise to lose weight** or suddenly become "fit"; instead, exercise at a mild to moderate level, and if you don't have a regular exercise routine, consult your doctor before starting anything new.

★ **Start slowly and build up** – 15-20 minutes at a time, three days a week, is plenty for beginners.

★ **Never exercise past the point** where you can't talk, or where you experience any discomfort.

★ **Keep yourself well hydrated,** stopping for sips of water as you go.

★ **Some activities should definitely be** avoided, including high-risk sports such as horse-riding, downhill skiing, snowboarding, water-skiing, and scuba diving. Weight-lifting and other exercises that involve standing in one place for longer periods can decrease the flow of blood to your baby.

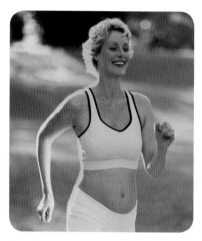

Running and jogging These are fine during early pregnancy, if you've done them before. Wear a pair of supportive trainers, and never push yourself too hard. Listen to your body and if you become very tired, stop.

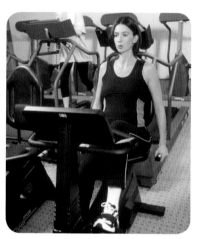

Cycling A good aerobic exercise, cycling builds stamina and strengthens leg muscles. The bike also supports your weight, but remember that you should never exercise too hard during pregnancy.

TOP TIP

Experts recommend that healthy pregnant women should aim for at least 150 minutes (about 2½ hours) of low-impact aerobic exercise every week.

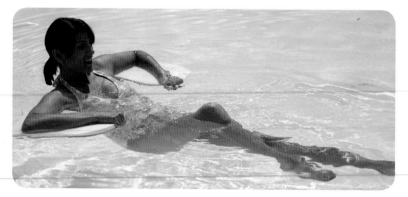

Swimming This is an ideal form of exercise during pregnancy, not only because it is aerobic and supports your weight, but it will also help you to relax. Swimming allows you to remain fit and supple without putting pressure on your joints. If you aren't a regular swimmer and find it hard work, why not consider an aquaerobics class designed for pregnancy?

Strengthening and toning

You don't have to leave your home to keep fit as even a little regular stretching can help to keep you in good shape for the months to come as your bump increases in size and weight. There's no doubt, too, that staying toned can help to make your labour that much easier.

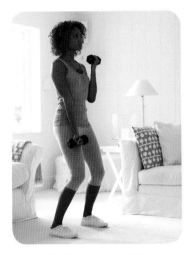

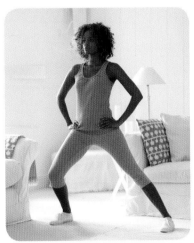

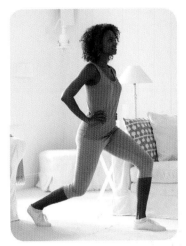

1 **Use light hand weights** designed for home use to stay supple. Heavy weights are not recommended during pregnancy.

2 **Gently stretching** your pelvis can help to support your growing abdomen. Strong pelvic muscles can also mean a shorter labour.

3 **Forward lunges** strengthen the muscles in your lower body and will help them to deal with the growing demands of pregnancy.

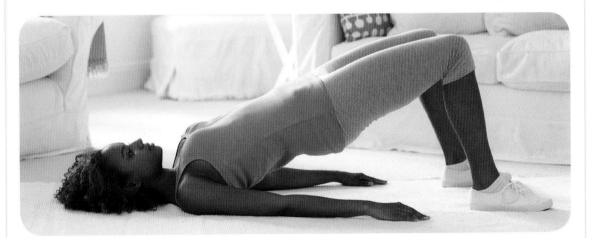

4 **The "bridge" exercise strengthens** your bottom, hamstrings, and inner thighs, and helps to build strength in your lower body. Doing this simple lift regularly can also help to prevent back pain, by strengthening the muscles that support your spine. This exercise is safe until the end of the second trimester, but always stop if you experience any discomfort.

Yoga and Pilates

Yoga and Pilates are ideal for pregnancy because they do not place undue pressure on your changing body, and offer all of the benefits of regular exercise. You'll experience improved flexibility, balance, and stamina, too.

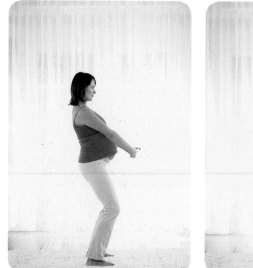
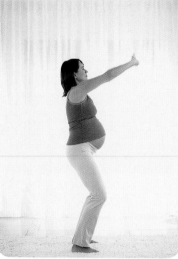
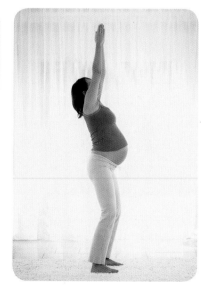

1 **"Salute to the sun"** can be practised throughout pregnancy, for as long as you feel comfortable. Stand with your feet apart, palms together, thumbs facing in.

2 **Inhale deeply** while you slowly raise your hands over your head, keeping your arms straight and your hands together as you do so.

3 **With your arms** up over your head, bend back very gently, while tightening your buttocks. Hold this pose for about three seconds.

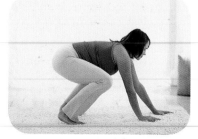
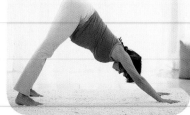
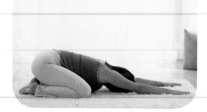

4 **Slowly exhale** and gently bend forward, slightly bending your knees for comfort, until your fingers touch the floor outside your feet.

5 **Inhale, and then exhale** again. Support your weight on your palms and toes, and straighten both legs so that you form a triangle with the floor.

6 **Slowly exhale,** bend both knees to the floor, bend your body with your hips in the air, then lower your chest and forehead to the floor.

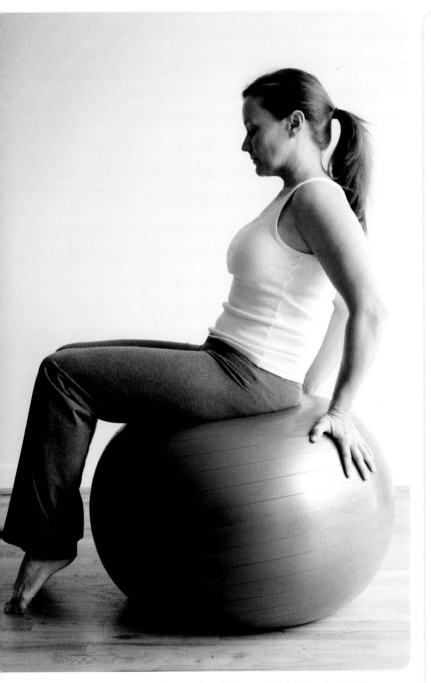

Pilates is ideal for pregnancy It strengthens both your abdominal and pelvic-floor muscles, without placing strain on your joints or your back. A Pilates exercise ball can be used under the supervision of an accredited instructor.

Why yoga and Pilates?

Both of these exercises can be undertaken at home, but if you've never done Pilates or yoga before look for a special antenatal class, or an instructor who can give you one-to-one attention.

Benefits Like all forms of exercise, these two disciplines will help you to maintain a healthy weight, promote restful sleep, reduce tension, encourage healthy circulation and digestion, help to speed up your labour, and get the endorphins flowing – the feel-good hormones that lift your mood and relieve pain. Even better, they strengthen and tone those muscles that will help to support the weight of your growing baby. Standing positions focus on achieving core stability, by strengthening the back and abdominal muscles.

Why yoga? A recent study found that women who practise yoga have a reduced risk of developing high blood pressure during pregnancy, and also going into premature labour. Yoga also encourages you to focus on your breathing, which can be a useful aid during labour.

Why Pilates? Pilates incorporates pelvic floor exercises (see pp.30–31), which are essential during pregnancy, as well as strengthening the core muscles, improving posture and circulation. You should have a more comfortable pregnancy and delivery when these muscles are toned. The exercises can be useful during labour, too, keeping you focused and mobile.

Your pelvic floor

The pelvic floor is a sling of muscles that forms the base of your pelvis and supports your uterus, bowels, and bladder. Exercising these muscles keeps them toned and makes you aware of them, so they can be relaxed during labour.

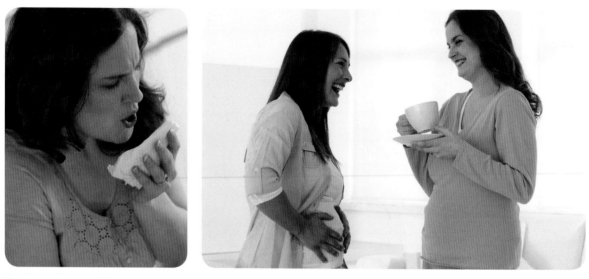

Coughs and sneezes Even these can prove to be too much of a strain for your pelvic floor if you don't keep the muscles toned.

Laughter Leaking a little urine when you laugh is perfectly normal during pregnancy, as your pelvic floor is under tremendous pressure from the weight of your uterus. If you exercise these muscles regularly, things should return to normal shortly after the birth.

Exercise techniques

With pelvic floor exercises, try to remember that it should be an "upward" and "inward" contraction, not a feeling of bearing down. Check that you are doing them correctly by putting your hand on your abdomen and buttocks, to be sure that you can feel your tummy, thighs, or buttocks moving.

"Slow" exercise This is the first of two exercises to work the two types of pelvic floor muscles. Slowly bring up your pelvic floor by contracting the muscles. Hold it for a count of five and then gently let it down again. You may find it easier to practise while sitting on a kitchen chair because you can actually feel the muscles as they rise and fall against the chair.

Work at this, several times a day, until you can hold the count for 15. You may lose control part way through but if so, start again, and perhaps try doing them while lying down to reduce the effect of gravity.

"Fast" exercise The second exercise involves quick tightening and releasing of the muscles in the pelvic floor. As quickly as you can, tighten and then release the muscles. Do this about 30 times.

A session This should comprise two sets of "slow" exercises and two sets of "fast" exercises. Take a minute's break in between each set. The most important thing is to remember to do both of the exercises several times a day.

Why your pelvic floor is important

During pregnancy, the weight of your baby and everything else required to sustain her life in the womb places enormous pressure on your pelvic floor muscles.

Labour benefits There is evidence to suggest that strong pelvic floor muscles can encourage a speedier labour and delivery, and, after the birth, help your perineum to heal. In fact, a strong set of these muscles can help to make the "pushing" second stage of labour (see pp.114-15) much more efficient, even if you have an epidural.

After the birth It's extremely important to keep these muscles toned to prevent a host of different problems. A strong pelvic floor helps to prevent stress incontinence (a slight leaking of urine when you cough or laugh). More seriously, it can also help to lessen the risk of prolapse, which occurs when your uterus slips down into your vagina.

What not to do When you practise the exercises, bear in mind the following: don't hold your breath (you should be able to keep up a conversation); don't tighten your tummy, thigh or buttock muscles; and don't squeeze your legs together. It may sound daunting, but since excess weight, hormonal changes, age, and abdominal surgery all affect this area, pelvic floor exercises should be practised for life.

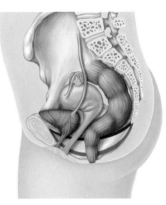

The muscles Pregnancy and birth inevitably affect the strength of your pelvic floor, the sling of muscles (outlined in purple) that support your pelvic organs.

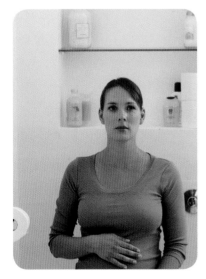

Feel the difference Empty your bladder before you begin your exercises. If you feel like going again afterwards, you are probably doing the exercises correctly. You may have heard that stopping your urine in mid-stream can help you locate the muscles but don't try this – it can push urine back up into the bladder and lead to infections.

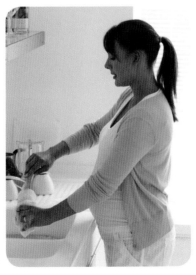

Multi-tasking Pelvic floor exercises, also known as "Kegels" after the doctor who designed them in the 1940s, can be undertaken anytime, anywhere. Get into the habit of doing a few sets while you are doing mundane tasks such as washing up. Remember them also while you're watching television or simply sitting at your desk.

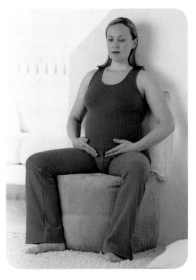

Don't forget Try to make a regular time for your pelvic floor exercises so you remember to do them. You could combine them with some yoga and stretching routines, but even if you just stick to the pelvic floor sets (see left) several times a day, you'll be gaining valuable health benefits for labour and the future.

A good night's sleep

Restful sleep can seem an elusive commodity, particularly as your pregnancy progresses; however, it's important to get as much as you can. Not only will it improve your mood and your overall energy levels, but you'll cope much better with your labour if you are well rested.

Feeling tired in the first trimester

In the first trimester, your body is busy developing both baby and placenta – no wonder you're tired!

New growth Fatigue is extremely common in the first few months of pregnancy, as you begin to adjust to the physical and emotional demands. It's worth remembering that you are effectively "growing" and developing a new human being in just nine months, so your body is hard at work nurturing this process.

Slow down Being tired is your body's way of telling you to ease up. Ideally, you need at least eight hours' sleep a night, so if you are used to working hard all day, preparing an evening meal, and socializing, too, you may not be getting all you need.

Well watered If you have reduced your caffeine consumption, fatigue can occur when you don't have that coffee/cola buzz. You may also be drinking insufficient water, so be sure to drink at least eight glasses a day.

Getting better This early fatigue will soon pass, and as you enter the second trimester, your energy levels will improve dramatically.

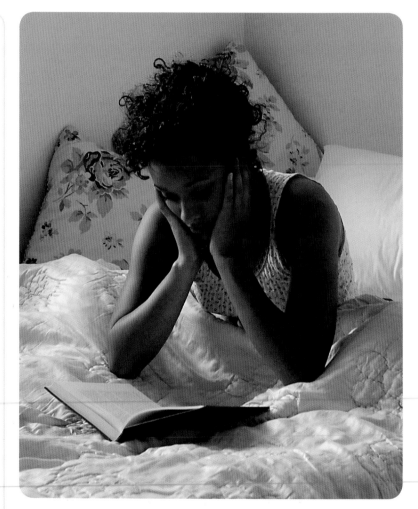

Take time to unwind before bed Even if you can't get to sleep, rest is important during pregnancy. Try to get yourself to bed early and relax until you drift off. The environment in which you sleep is particularly important now, which means making sure your bedroom is quiet and a comfortable temperature, and that you are cosy in bed.

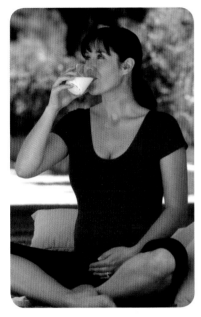

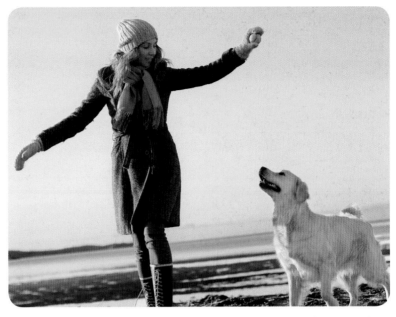

A glass of milk before bed Milk and dairy products, eggs, and tuna, are great sources of the amino acid tryptophan, which encourages restful sleep.

Regular exercise This will help to make sure that you are physically tired enough to sleep and will also help to reduce the impact of any stress you are experiencing. Get at least 30 minutes a day, preferably out in the fresh air if you can. Walking the dog or leaving the car behind for short errands are easy ways to achieve this.

Sleeping positions

As your pregnancy progresses, you may have to adjust your usual sleeping position. There are a few different positions that may help you to get a better night's sleep. Invest in some good, firm pillows that will help to support your growing bump and make you feel more comfortable.

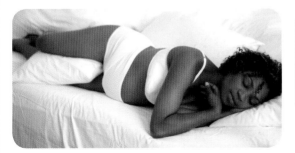

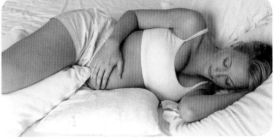

Using pillows As your bump gets bigger and heavier, try placing a pillow between your legs to provide support for your hips. You can also wedge a pillow under your lower back to relieve pressure in that area. You may need to change these around a little to find a comfortable position as your bump gets bigger.

Sleep on your left side You might find that sleeping on your left side is more comfortable. This will relieve pressure on the major blood vessels that supply oxygen and nutrients to your baby. Experiment with pillows: try using one to support your bump comfortably and another to gently lift your thigh and knee.

When you can't sleep

Sleep problems can be frustrating and debilitating, particularly when you need to be well rested for your impending birth and life with your new baby.

Sleep solutions

★ Eat tryptophan-rich foods before bed (see p.33) for restful sleep.

★ Avoid caffeine and other stimulants, which can discourage sleep and make you feel restless and anxious.

★ A warm cup of chamomile tea before bedtime can relax you so that you can drift off more easily.

★ Make sure you aren't too hot; you may wish to use a separate set of sheets and blankets so that you can peel off layers when you feel uncomfortable, without waking your partner.

★ If heartburn is keeping you awake, try sleeping with your body upright on a nest of pillows. Another good trick is to eat a slice of fresh pineapple after your main meal, which helps to neutralize the acid.

★ Relax. If you begin to panic that you'll never get to sleep, you probably won't. A poor night's sleep can be disruptive and exhausting, but it's not the end of the world. You can catch up later.

★ Try doing some relaxation exercises. Starting with your toes, tighten and then relax the muscles in your body. Continue all the way up your legs, abdomen, chest, arms, and finally your face.

★ Ask your partner to give you a massage, which can ease tension that could be preventing restful sleep.

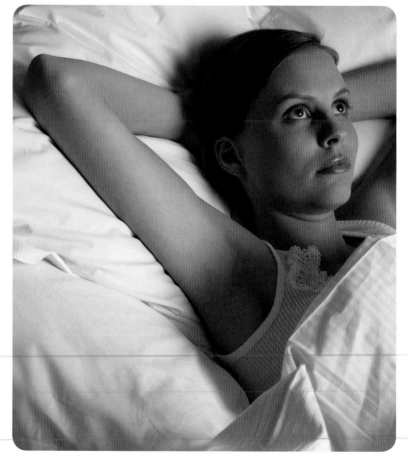

Lying awake If, like many women, you experience sleeplessness during pregnancy, try to make sure that you get plenty of fresh air and exercise and that you are eating a healthy diet that includes slow-release carbohydrates. Some women have "restless legs syndrome", in which their legs feel "twitchy" in bed. If you find this is a problem, try raising your feet on a pillow.

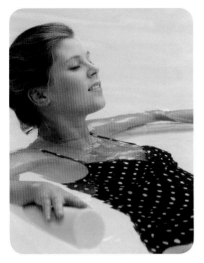 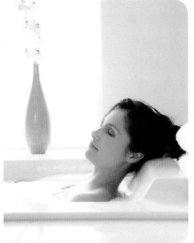 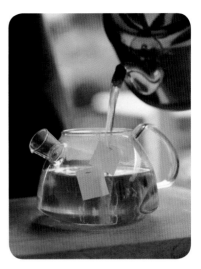

Exercise to sleep Swimming will both tire and relax you. It also allows you to exercise without putting pressure on your joints, so you are less likely to have back and other aches and pains during the night.

Run a bath Take a warm, but not hot, bath just before bedtime, and consider adding a few drops of lavender essential oil, which can soothe and relax you. Lie back and allow the water to support your growing bump.

Chamomile tea If you find yourself lying awake, try drinking a cup of warm chamomile tea, but don't overdo it, or you may find that frequent trips to the bathroom will be keeping you awake instead.

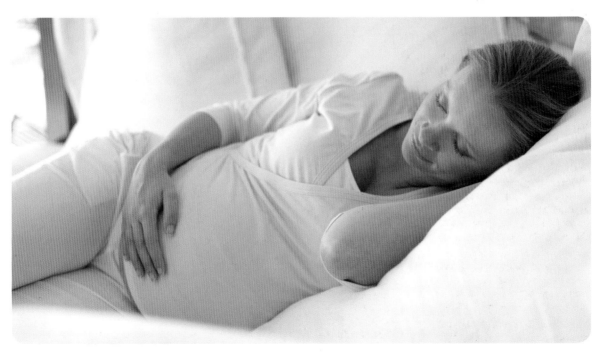

Take naps If you aren't getting enough sleep at night-time, try to nap during the day. The best advice is to listen to your body, and sleep when you are tired. A nap may be just what you need to revive you, and allow you to get through the remainder of the day.

Emotional symptoms

It's not unusual to experience extreme highs and lows, as your body adjusts to the changing hormones that accompany pregnancy. Add to this the fact that your life is about to change dramatically, and it's not surprising that your emotions are less stable and your moods tend to swing in all directions.

Stay balanced

Finding a balance between the highs and lows of pregnancy will help you to feel more in control, and less concerned that your emotions will get the better of you. The following tips will help:

★ Try to remember that experiencing emotional ups and downs is completely normal, and most common during the first and third trimesters.

★ Eat regular, healthy meals to keep your blood-sugar levels stable; this will help to even out your moods.

★ Get plenty of restful sleep, taking naps as and when you need to. Fatigue and exhaustion can quickly make you irritable and moody.

★ Exercise not only increases the "feel-good" hormones in your body, but also helps to reduce stress and encourage restful sleep. All of these impact on your emotional wellbeing.

★ Ask your friends and family for support, and don't be afraid to explain how you are feeling.

★ Take the pressure off; some women race towards the end of their pregnancies, fitting in as much as possible. Pregnancy isn't a race or a destination, and it really doesn't matter if you don't have absolutely everything organized in advance.

★ Take time for a little pampering; treats are guaranteed to lift your spirits, particularly if your changing body is making you feel a little ungainly.

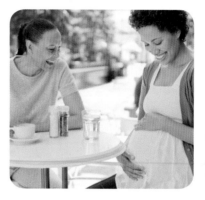

Your mood It is a common feature of pregnancy to feel elated and overwhelmed with happiness at times, but you may find that your moods shift dramatically for no apparent reason. Enjoy the highs, and use these moments to get on with enjoyable activities.

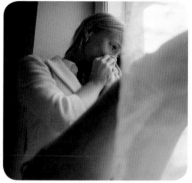

Tearfulness This is not just normal, but to be expected. The hormone changes taking place can make you weepy, but it's worth noting that this can be a symptom of depression, so talk to your midwife if it's happening regularly.

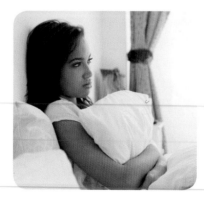

Feeling blue If you are feeling low, create a little time for yourself. If you are well rested and able to relax, you'll be much less likely to suffer from both the emotional and physical symptoms of pregnancy.

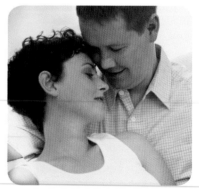

Make time to talk Talking things through regularly with your partner can help to ease the pressure and deal with some of the anxieties and concerns that are common for both partners to experience.

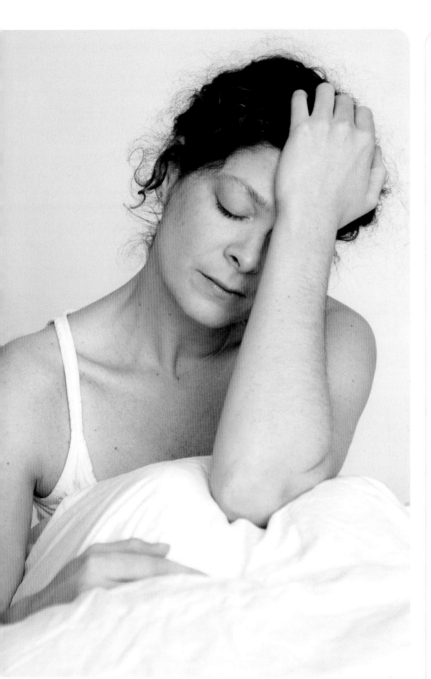

A common problem Long periods of depression, tearfulness, or anxiety can be a sign of antenatal depression (see right), which is believed to be a result of the hormonal shifts of pregnancy, combined with stress. With more women struggling to juggle jobs and pregnancy, it's not surprising that this condition is becoming more common.

Antenatal depression

Although not as commonly known as postnatal depression, this condition can be treated so don't be afraid to ask for help.

Under diagnosed Up to 25 per cent of women experience some depression in pregnancy, and about half of those will suffer from a diagnosable condition, known as "antenatal depression". Because it is natural to feel blue during pregnancy, this condition is often under diagnosed, or considered to be something temporary. However, being aware of the symptoms and getting help can make sure that you get the support and treatment you need to feel better.

Symptoms You may be suffering from antenatal depression if you experience some of the following symptoms for more than two weeks:
★ Difficulty sleeping (or even sleeping too much).
★ Regular crying.
★ Loss of interest or pleasure in activities you usually enjoy.
★ Feelings of guilt or worthlessness.
★ Loss of energy and noticeable difficulty concentrating.
★ Changes in appetite and normal eating patterns.
★ Feeling restless or irritable.
★ Feeling sad and hopeless.
★ Withdrawing from your partner, family, and friends.
★ Thoughts or ideas about suicide.

Treatment There are different types of therapies and medication (some anti-depressants are considered safe during pregnancy) that can help. Speak to your midwife or GP for advice.

Physical symptoms

Although many women experience virtually no symptoms at all, the most debilitating ones, such as morning sickness, tend to occur early in pregnancy, as your body adjusts to hormonal changes. Most will pass, and with the help of a few tried-and-tested tips, you can sail through your pregnancy with ease.

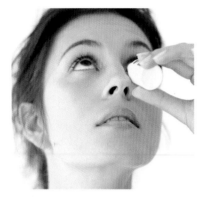

Eye problems Your eyes may be drier than usual, or you may experience sensitivity to light, itching, or excessive watering due to a fall in male hormones (androgens). If you wear contact lenses, you may wish to switch back to glasses or ask your GP for eye drops.

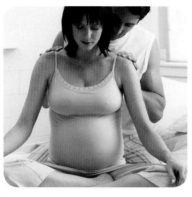

Back pain The extra weight of your baby as well as softening ligaments can cause back pain, particularly in your lower back. Good posture will keep your backbone aligned properly and regular massage will loosen any tension and ease discomfort.

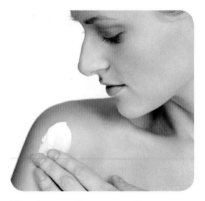

Skin changes You may experience spots and dry, dull, or blotchy skin during pregnancy. Rest assured that things will return to normal once you've given birth; in the meantime, drink plenty of water and use a light moisturiser.

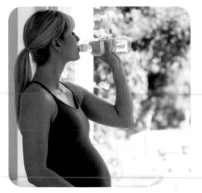

Headaches and constipation Drinking plenty of water throughout the day is the best way to prevent both of these. Your fluid needs increase during pregnancy, so carry a bottle of water in your bag.

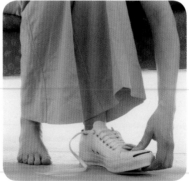

Swelling During pregnancy more water is collected in the body, which causes swelling or "oedema", particularly in the legs and feet. To counter this, try to put your feet up as often as possible throughout the day.

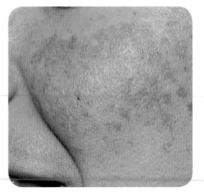

Pigmentation marks These can appear at any stage of pregnancy, and can be distressing for some women. Protect your skin with a good sunscreen, and remember that marks will fade after your baby is born.

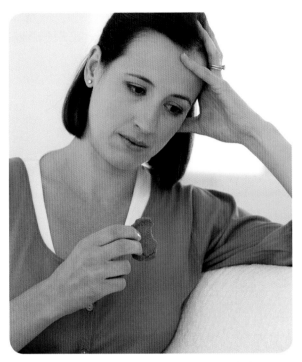

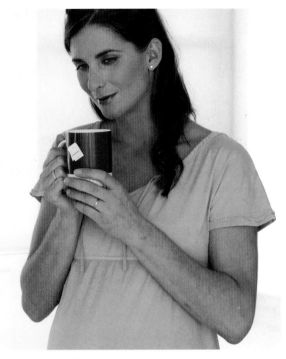

Ginger If you are feeling nauseous, try eating ginger (fresh, preserved, or even in biscuit form) to ease the symptoms and settle your stomach. Eating little and often can also help to balance your blood sugar, which can make you feel a little better.

Chamomile tea This can help to ease nausea by working directly on your digestive system. It will also help to keep you hydrated, which may be a problem if you are vomiting. You can also try a vitamin B_6 supplement (see below), as a deficiency may be making things worse.

Coping with morning sickness

Morning sickness can be one of the most debilitating symptoms of pregnancy, and can occur well after the morning has passed. In most women, symptoms are worse in the first trimester, settling down once hormone levels stabilize. Here are a few steps you can take to ease symptoms:

★ Symptoms are often worse when you are hungry, so eat little and often to stabilize your blood-sugar.

★ Dry biscuits seem to help ease nausea in many cases.

★ Drink plenty of water – if you are vomiting regularly dehydration can make the nausea worse.

★ Eat a little first thing in the morning, even before you get out of bed.

★ Avoid fatty foods and junk foods, which seem to make symptoms worse.

★ Invest in motion-sickness wrist bands; strap them onto your wrists so that the plastic button presses against an acupressure point on your inside wrist. Many women have found these to be very helpful in easing nausea and vomiting.

★ Get plenty of sleep and take regular rests, which can make a big difference to the way you feel.

★ Wear comfortable clothing; you may find that anything tight around your neck or abdomen can make you feel worse.

★ Consider taking a supplement of vitamin B_6, which has been shown to be deficient in many cases of morning sickness. Take 50mg per day, or increase your intake of B_6-rich foods, such as poultry, pork, eggs, whole grain cereals, milk and soya beans.

★ Try to remember that almost all cases pass by the end of the first trimester, when your hormones settle down.

★ If your symptoms are severe, debilitating, and do not improve, your doctor may prescribe an anti-emetic, which is an anti-sickness medicine that is effective in the short term.

When to see your doctor

It's common to experience a multitude of symptoms during pregnancy, including unexpected twinges and grumbling discomfort. However, if they continue, see a doctor.

See your doctor if:

★ Any illness lasts longer than 48 hours, including vomiting, diarrhoea, and even colds or flu.

★ You have a high temperature.

★ You experience vision problems or extreme headaches.

★ Your baby stops moving.

★ You experience anxiety or confusion with a racing heart or rapid breathing.

★ You pass any clots of pink, grey, or red material.

★ There is any sudden swelling of your face or hands.

★ You experience severe abdominal pain, stabbing pains, or cramping.

★ You find it difficult to breathe or suffer from chest pain.

★ Urinating is painful.

★ Your skin becomes extremely itchy.

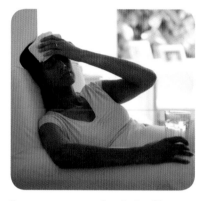

Frequent or severe headaches You should be seen immediately by a doctor; they can indicate dangerous complications, such as pre-eclampsia.

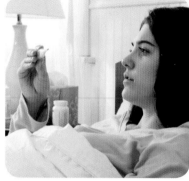

Infectious diseases If you feel ill and have been in contact with an infectious disease that might harm your unborn baby, contact your doctor or midwife for advice immediately.

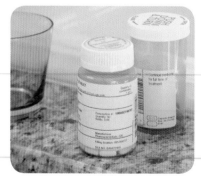

Medication If you were taking any medication before you became pregnant, talk to your doctor about it. Your dosages or drugs may need to be changed.

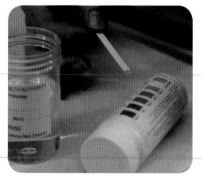

Gestational diabetes If you are thought to be at risk of developing this condition (see p.58), your urine will be tested for sugar at your antenatal appointments.

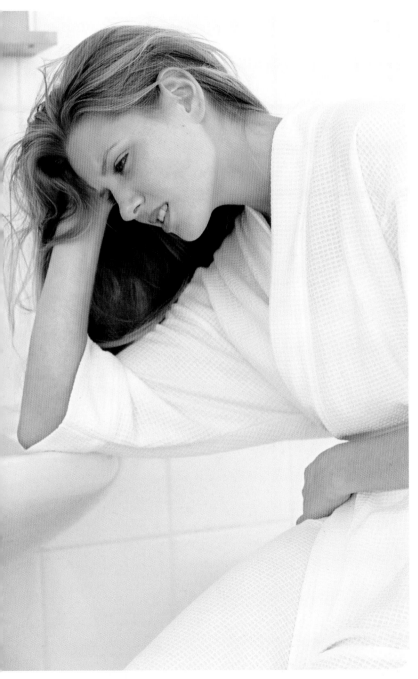

Mild cramping Some mild cramping in pregnancy is completely normal but any severe cramping or sharp, stabbing pains should be reported to your doctor as soon as possible, particularly if they are accompanied by any bleeding.

Ectopic pregnancies

An ectopic pregnancy occurs when a fertilized egg becomes established in your fallopian tube. It is potentially life-threatening and will require urgent medical attention. Ectopic pregnancies are not viable.

What happens? It is thought that the fertilized egg becomes "caught" while progressing down the fallopian tube. In this case the baby continues to grow inside the tube where it can cause the tube to burst, or severely damage it. If a negative pregnancy test follows a positive one, there is a possibility that your pregnancy is ectopic.

Symptoms include:
★ One-sided pain in your tummy.
★ Shoulder-tip pain; typical of ectopic pregnancies, this affects the point where your shoulder ends and your arm starts. It may be due to internal bleeding irritating the diaphragm when you breathe in and out.
★ Painful bowel movements or pain on urination.
★ Feeling light-headed or faint.
★ An unusual period, with dark, watery, or slight bleeding.

Diagnosing It can often be difficult for doctors to reach a diagnosis because symptoms can occur from about three weeks after conception until 12 weeks or later. What's more, there can be other causes for many of the symptoms.

What to do If you believe you are pregnant, and experience any of the symptoms, go to your local accident and emergency unit.

Balancing pregnancy and work

No matter how career-orientated you are, becoming pregnant does involve slowing down a little. Aim to establish a healthy balance between a satisfying work life, and a home life that can grow in importance.

Hazards at work

It is completely safe to continue working in most jobs and companies; however, it is important to be aware of the potential risks to you and/or your baby. You should avoid:

★ **Awkward spaces** and work stations.

★ **Working with animals,** whose waste, bodies, and surroundings may carry *E. coli*, tulareanaemia, toxoplasmosis, histoplasmosis, and other disease-causing organisms.

★ **Chemicals,** such as those used in medical, dental, or pharmaceutical occupations, plus painting, cleaning, farming, dry-cleaning, gardening, pest-control, carpet-cleaning, and more. Check the safety data on every chemical with which you come into contact.

★ **Food hazards,** such as listeria, *E. coli*, and salmonella, which can be acquired by handling raw food.

★ **Heavy lifting.**

★ **Long hours** of standing or sitting.

★ **Slippery floors.**

★ **Radiation,** from repeated exposure to x-rays, for example.

★ **Viral hazards,** particularly in medical environments or even childcare facilities, where you may come into contact with viruses, including childhood illnesses such as Rubella (see p.57), which may be harmful to your unborn baby.

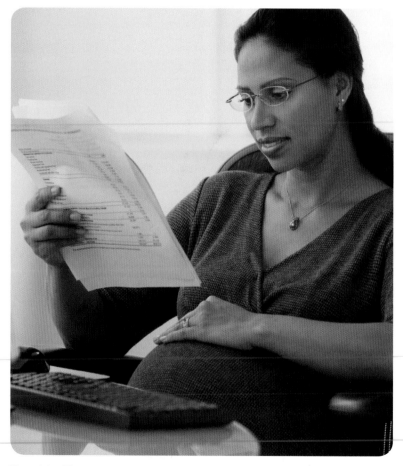

Your rights There are very strict guidelines supporting your rights during pregnancy, and you will also be entitled to a variety of benefits. It's always a good idea to investigate what's on offer, so you know where you stand. The most important thing to remember is that pregnancy does not make you incompetent, and you cannot be sacked for being pregnant.

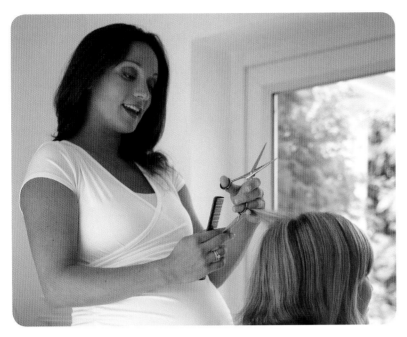

Taking it easy

Take a step back and get the rest and relaxation you need to stay on top and control potentially harmful stress.

Recharge your batteries Take occasional extra breaks, or work shorter hours if that's on offer. But play it carefully. Make sure you keep up with your work, and don't demand special attention; how you behave greatly influences how others will treat you.

Be organized Being prepared during working hours will help you to remain professional. Keep a comfortable pair of shoes under your desk. Eat healthy snacks and drink plenty of water to keep you going. Keep a notebook listing ongoing projects in case you need to hand them over to colleagues early.

Getting the best out of your day If you stand for long periods or have a stressful job, take regular breaks. You may also find that you feel more in control of things if you make productive use of your lunch hours, to fit in tasks that need to be completed before your baby arrives.

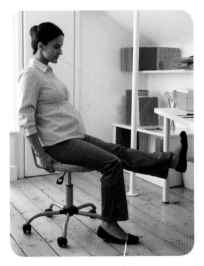

Be comfortable Take time to do a few stretching exercises, and keep your feet up on a footstool as often as you can. Not only will this prevent swelling, but it can help you to feel more comfortable and relaxed.

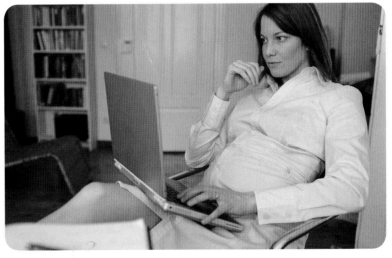

A healthy balance If you are used to taking work home and allowing your job to take over your life, it's time to make a few adjustments. Life with a baby will simply not allow this approach to work, and you will need to find a healthier work-life balance. It's a good idea to establish with your employer at the outset how your priorities will be changing, and what you feel you can realistically offer in your new circumstances.

Your developing body

It's almost impossible to believe that your body can adapt and change to create a whole new life in just nine short months. Not only will your shape change dramatically over this period, but you'll notice a host of other transformations as well, as your body prepares to deliver your new baby to the world, and then nourish her for the months to come.

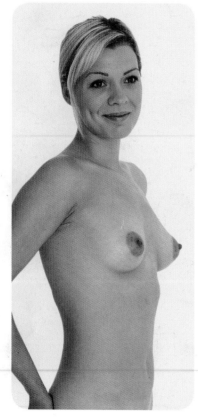 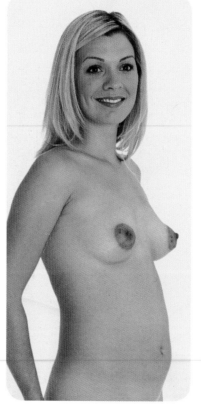 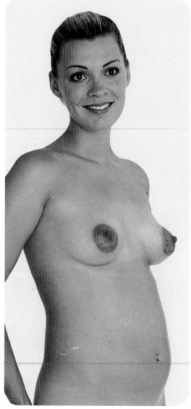

8 weeks Your shape will not have changed dramatically by eight weeks, although some women report a gentle rounding of the abdomen. Your breasts may be tender, and you may experience some nausea, urinary frequency, and cravings, as well as an increase in vaginal discharge. You may also have some mild, period-like cramping.

16 weeks Because your placenta has taken over production of pregnancy hormones, you will feel less emotional and any morning sickness may have waned. Your heart will be beating more rapidly because of the extra volume of blood in your body. Your breasts will have increased in size, and feel fuller and more tender.

20 weeks Your uterus has now expanded to reach your navel, and you will be showing more. You may begin to feel your baby move. It's very common to have to urinate frequently as your kidneys work harder. Your breasts will begin to feel much fuller and heavier, your areolas will darken, and you may need to invest in a maternity bra.

Weight gain in pregnancy

No matter how fit you are, or how well you eat, you will gain weight in pregnancy, and this is to be encouraged. On average, most women will put on 10–12.5kg (22–28lb) over nine months.

★ It is usual to gain about 1.8kg (4lb) in the first trimester, about 6.4kg (14lb) in the second, and about 4.6kg (10lb) in the third. However, these are average numbers and depend on your starting weight, and the size of your baby. Mums-to-be of twins can expect to put on between 18.2 and 22.7kg (40 and 50lb).

★ The weight you gain will be made up of the weight of your baby, the placenta, extra fluid, increased blood, amniotic fluid, your uterus, fat deposits, and increased breast size.

★ Most importantly, eat well and take some gentle exercise.

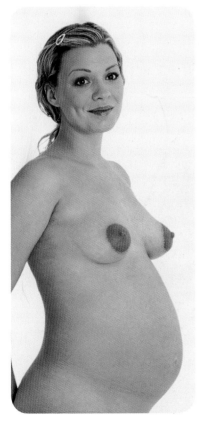

28 weeks As you enter your last trimester, you may experience back pain, oedema, and sleep difficulties. Your abdomen will grow rapidly, and you may be able to see your baby's kicks. Place your hand on your abdomen and feel your baby move towards it. Your joints will become looser as your body prepares for the birth.

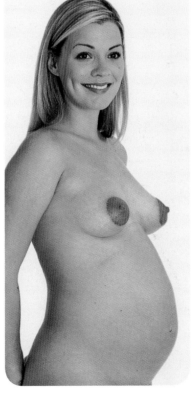

32 weeks Your abdomen will be very prominent now. You may have a linea nigra, (see p.46) and perhaps some stretch marks. You may also find that you are rather uncomfortable, tiring easily and having trouble sleeping. As your baby descends into your pelvis, you may find breathing easier, but have to urinate more frequently.

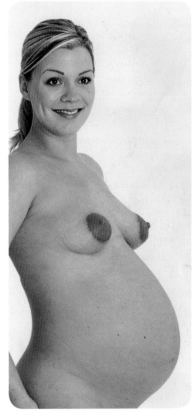

40 weeks Your uterus will now measure about 40cm (16in) from your pubic bone. You may have more frequent and painful practice contractions. You might also have a "show", which means that the plug of jelly-like mucus that sealed your womb against infection is discharged as your cervix begins to dilate for labour.

Physical changes

As your pregnancy progresses, the physical changes to your body will become more pronounced, and you may need new clothes to accommodate your growing size. A professionally fitted maternity bra is a must from mid-pregnancy, and you may need to replace it a few months later.

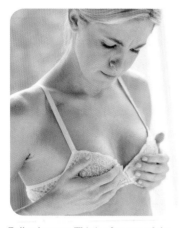

Fuller breasts This is often one of the first signs of pregnancy. Your nipples may also become larger and darker, and you may notice Montgomery's tubercles (small white bumps on your areolas).

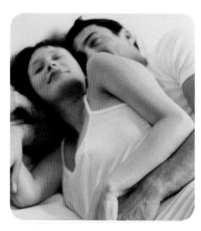

Your libido Your sex drive is largely guided by your hormones, so expect fluctuations. It may wax and wane throughout pregnancy; you may feel glowing, and then find that fatigue takes sex firmly off the menu.

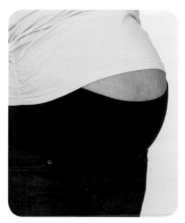

Your abdomen It could begin to expand from as early as eight weeks, although the 16th week or so is usual for many women. Remind yourself that it's all worth it to have your new baby.

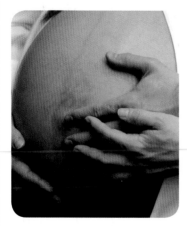

The linea nigra This is a dark, vertical line that can appear between your navel and your pubic area. Caused by the same pregnancy hormones that darken your areolas, it will disappear after birth.

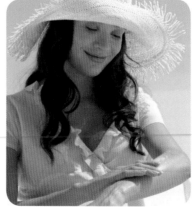

Skin sensitivity As your skin changes throughout pregnancy, you may find that it is more sensitive to the sun, and prone to freckling and burning. Always moisturize and wear a good sunscreen.

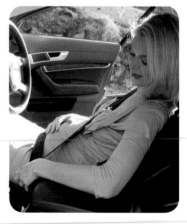

Feeling unwieldy There's no doubt that you'll feel cumbersome from time to time, and you'll need to learn to accommodate your new clumsiness, expanded girth, and lack of balance.

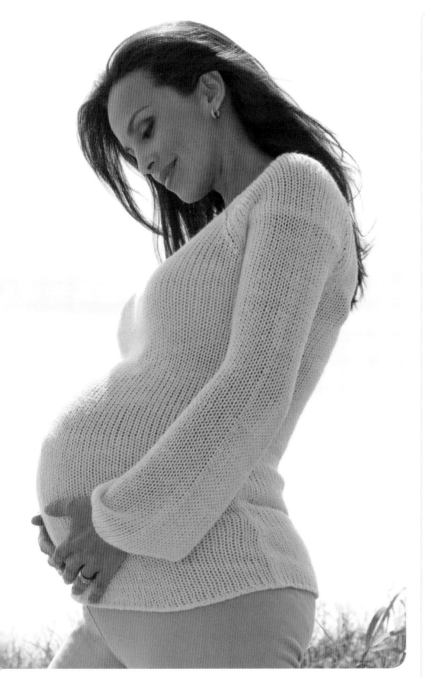

Your maternity wardrobe

Although you can undoubtedly "make do and mend" for a good proportion of your pregnancy, there are a few essentials you will need to see you through to delivery day:

★ Maternity clothing is specially designed to accommodate a large and growing bump; larger-sized normal clothing will simply be too tight and loose in the wrong places.

★ Start with a few items and add pieces as you need them. You'll be wearing the same maternity clothes for at least four or five months.

★ Invest in two good-quality maternity bras to accommodate your changing size, and don't be surprised if they need to be replaced in a few months' time.

★ Don't hesitate to accept offers of maternity clothes from friends and relatives; even if they are not right for your office dress code, wearing them at home will allow you to spend a little more on work clothing.

★ You can also purchase a "belly band", which is designed to fill the gap between skirts or trousers and your usual tops, as your waist expands.

★ For the office, purchase a few good pieces of neutral, simply shaped, basic but smart garments, and accessorize them with a variety of scarves and jewellery.

★ Don't forget your shoes. Your centre of gravity changes when you are pregnant, as your weight shifts forward, and high heels can be dangerous and uncomfortable. Look for elegant flats or low heels instead.

★ Finally, remember that looking great and being comfortable can help you to feel more confident about your growing size.

The "glow" One of the joys of pregnancy is the "glow" that seems to radiate from you, particularly during the second trimester. Your skin may become more luminous and your hair thicker. But don't be surprised if you also experience a few, less pleasant changes too.

Your growing baby

From the moment of conception, your baby will begin to grow and develop at an astonishing rate; in fact, he will be capable of wondrous new things almost every single day of your pregnancy. Keeping tabs on your baby's development can make your pregnancy even more exciting.

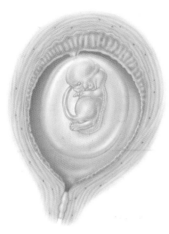

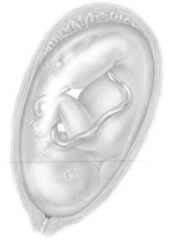

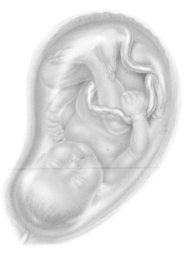

1st trimester (8 weeks) Your baby is now amazingly 10,000 times bigger than the size of the fertilized egg. His face is beginning to form, and his eyes are now visible under his skin. Your baby's spinal column is in place and his brain and bones are forming.

2nd trimester (28 weeks) All of your baby's organs are functioning apart from his lungs, which are still filled with amniotic fluid. His brain has reached a startling level of development, and his muscular and nervous systems are developing rapidly.

3rd trimester (40 weeks) Your full-term baby is in position for his birth, although he may not always be head down. Over the past few weeks his weight has increased by about 200g (8oz) per week. He will be starting to look plump.

Timeline

From the moment your egg is fertilized your body will undergo a massive series of changes, as the embryo grows and develops into a healthy, full-term baby.

1	2	3	4	5	6	7	8	9	10	11	12	13	14	15	16	17	18	19	20

★ First trimester   ★ Second trimester

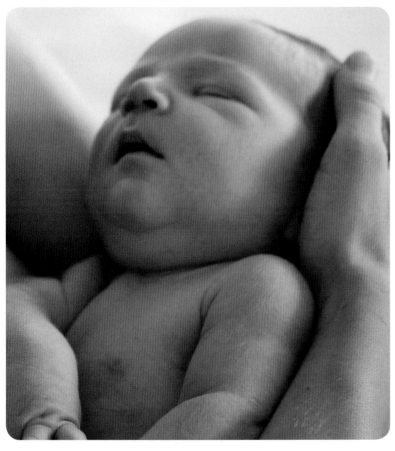

Your newborn baby He may or may not look exactly as you imagined, but at last all that waiting and wondering will be over. If you're lucky, it may be love at first sight, but if not, don't worry, you have a whole lifetime to get to know each other.

How big will your baby be?

Your baby's growth and development in the womb will be dramatic. Remember, however, that it's not his size, but position that can make birth more or less difficult.

Average figures At two weeks, he'll be less than a millimetre in length, but by the end of the first trimester, your baby will have grown to 10cm (3in) in length, and weigh around 45g (2oz). At 24 weeks, he'll have increased his weight to 650g (1lb 7oz) and measure about 30cm – nearly a foot long! When you are 28 weeks pregnant, your baby will top 1kg (2lb 3oz), and be 35cm (13in) long, and just four weeks later, he'll be 1.9kg (4lb 3oz) and 40.5cm (15in). Things then slow down a little and at full term, the average baby will weigh about 3.5kg (7lb 8oz) and be about 50cm (19in) long.

Your baby's size Your midwife will be able to give you an idea of how big your baby is likely to be once you are around 36 weeks.

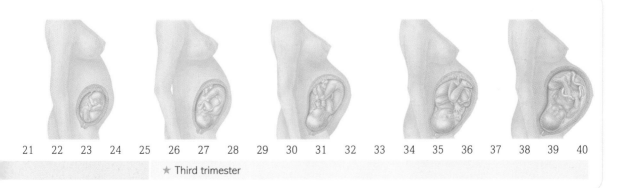

21 22 23 24 25 26 27 28 29 30 31 32 33 34 35 36 37 38 39 40

★ Third trimester

12 weeks Your baby is just over 5cm (2in) long from crown to bottom, and is already a recognizable human being. Although his head is relatively large, the rest of his body is catching up and is becoming straighter.

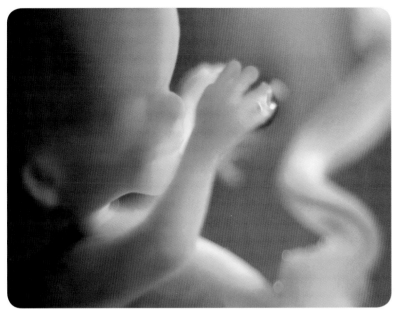

15 weeks He is now about 9–10cm (about 4in) long, and is covered by lanugo (fine hair). His face is much more human in appearance, although he has a wide mouth and a very small chin. The bridge of his nose is shallow and his eyes still dominate his face. He'll usually have his hands by his face, and will soon begin to think about sucking his thumb. It won't be long before you feel his movements.

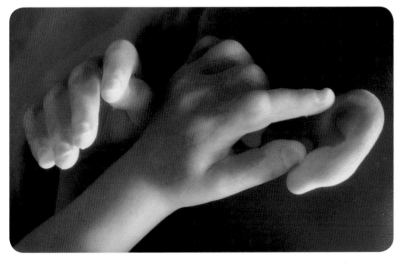

19 weeks Your baby has been experiencing rapid growth that now begins to slow down. He's about 18cm (at least 7in) from crown to bottom, and his legs are in proportion to his body. He is hearing sounds outside the womb, and will begin to respond to them. You may feel your baby moving, particularly when you lie down.

Going live

Your first scan will amaze you, as you see a very real baby alive and kicking in his comfortable home.

Boy or girl? At 20 weeks, the sex of your baby can clearly be seen, although if you do not wish to know, remember to tell the sonographer before they begin the scan.

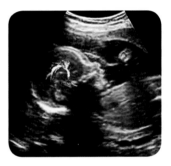

Your baby's features These will change little before his birth, and the profile on your scan photo is, in fact, a pretty clear representation of how your baby will look when he arrives.

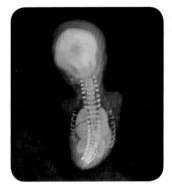

Your baby's spine This begins to develop from the fourth week of pregnancy, when he is smaller than the head of a pin. You will be able to see it clearly on your first scan.

51

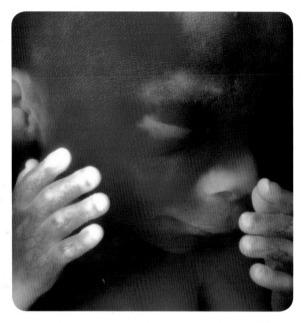

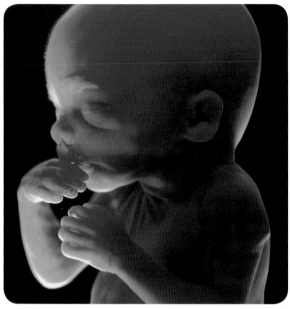

21 weeks By now, your baby's features are fully formed, and he looks almost exactly like a smaller version of the baby who will be delivered in four months' time. His hair is growing and the soft cartilage in his body is gradually hardening into bone.

24 weeks Your baby has grown dramatically, but is yet to fill out. He is now around 30cm (12in) from top to toe, and his organ systems – including his nervous, reproductive, circulatory, and digestive systems – are continuing to develop.

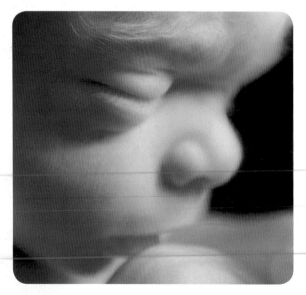

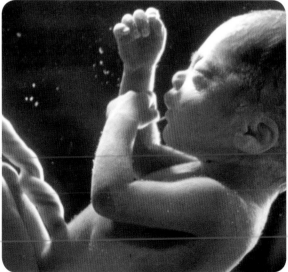

27 weeks Your baby's immune system and his lungs are beginning to mature. He has now laid down stores of fat and would have a good chance of surviving if he was born today.

37 weeks Conditions in the womb are becoming very cramped. He is now fully formed and begins to behave just like a newborn: sucking, sleeping, breathing, and even urinating.

40 weeks – full term Although you may now be experiencing some very strong and quite painful Braxton Hicks' contractions, the amniotic fluid that surrounds your baby ensures that he hardly notices these tightenings.

Your scans

Your first scan may not only offer an opportunity to catch your first glimpse of your baby, but it will also provide your doctor and midwife with important information about her overall health, growth, and development.

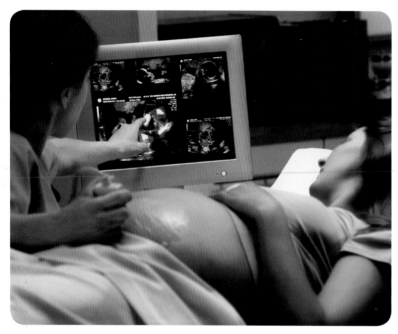

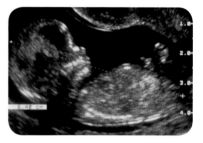

Scans Most women have two scans – at 10–14 weeks (above), and at 20 weeks. Women who have previously miscarried or bled may be offered one at six to 10 weeks, too.

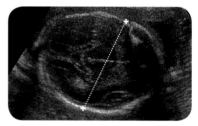

At hospital Your midwife will arrange for you to have a routine "dating scan" at around 10–14 weeks. Your baby (or babies, if there are more than one) will be measured from her head to her bottom (the crown-rump length), You may also have a nuchal translucency (NT) scan, which assesses the risk of Down's syndrome (see p.56).

The dating scan At the 10–14 week scan, the diameter of your baby's skull is measured to give an accurate idea of her age.

The importance of your scans

Not only is it now firmly established that seeing your baby in the womb reinforces the bonding process, but your midwife and doctor will also be aware of any potential problems early on.

★ Your dating scan is crucial to judge whether your baby's development and growth match your dates. It will also be used to check for multiple pregnancies as they will require extra antenatal attention.

★ Your 20-week scan will provide a full check of your baby. The biparietal diameter (the bones at the top of the skull) will be measured, as well as her head circumference, abdominal circumference,

and the length of her thigh bone. The sonographer will look for a cleft lip and possibly cleft palate as well as checking her spine, heart, stomach, kidneys, legs, arms, hands, feet, fingers, and toes.

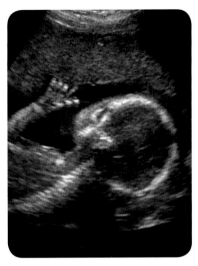

20-week scan This is known as an "anomaly" scan, and is designed to check your baby carefully for abnormalities. You may be able to see the sex of your baby on the scan, and the sonographer will also check the position of the placenta in your womb.

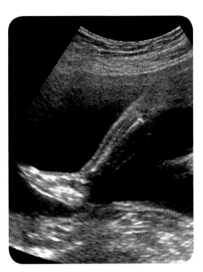

Checks At the 20-week scan, your baby will have her legs, arms, hands, feet, fingers, and toes examined. You will be able to see your baby's bones, and many of her organs. Your sonographer will also be checking that urine flows from the kidneys to the bladder.

3D scans

Most hospitals offer parents-to-be black and white photographs of their 2D scans, but some now also offer startlingly detailed 3D images, too.

3D scans These provide a sophisticated, three-dimensional view of your baby and her bones and organs so you can see her in great detail. Some hospitals use this type of scanning to encourage early bonding, but it can also provide a very accurate check for anomalies such as cleft palate or cleft lip.

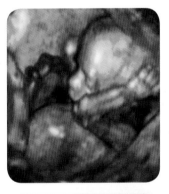

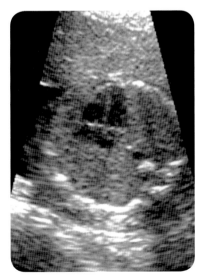

Your baby's heart This will be examined to check that the top two and bottom two chambers are the same size. The valves should open and close as your baby's heart beats and you may be able to see the blood vessels entering and leaving the heart.

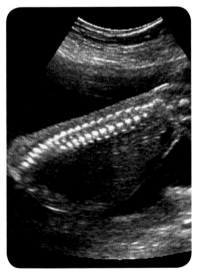

Your baby's spine Her spine will be checked in detail – both its length, and in cross-section. By doing so, the sonographer is trying to establish that all of the bones are aligned, and that your baby's skin fully covers her spine at the back.

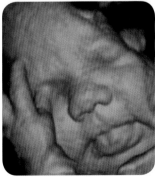

4D scans These are moving 3D images, showing your baby in action in her first "feature film".

Screening tests

Throughout your pregnancy, you will undergo a number of tests to establish your health and that of your baby. Some of these tests are optional, and your midwife or doctor will discuss the implications of having them done or declining them.

Tests you may have:

Your blood will be tested for:

★ Your blood group.

★ Your Rhesus status (whether you have a positive or negative blood type).

★ HIV.

★ Haemoglobin and ferritin levels.

★ Hepatitis B.

★ Rubella immunity.

★ Red cell blood abnormalities.

Screening tests:

★ Urine tests – if a risk is identified.

★ Blood pressure.

★ The "triple" or "quadruple" blood test (at 11–16 weeks) to check for hormones that could indicate spina bifida or Down's syndrome. Or you may be offered a combined NT scan (see right) and blood test.

Diagnostic tests: if screening tests suggest a high risk of Down's or other chromosomal abnormalities.

★ Chorionic villus sampling (CVS), in which tiny samples of the chorionic villi (from the placenta) are taken to check the genetic information they carry. Transvaginal CVS is done at 11–13 weeks, when a small tube is inserted through your cervix. Transabdominal CVS is usually done after 13 weeks, when a needle is inserted through your abdomen into your placenta.

★ Amniocentesis (see right).

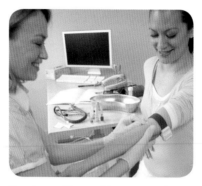

Blood tests These will be undertaken at, or shortly after, your booking appointment; the results will usually be ready when you have your next scheduled antenatal appointment, but your midwife or doctor will be in touch if there are any concerns.

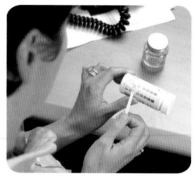

Urine tests Your urine will be tested at every appointment to check for the presence of protein (which could indicate pre-eclampsia) and urinary tract infections. If you are at risk of gestational diabetes (see p.58), your urine and blood will be tested for sugar.

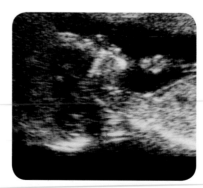

Nuchal translucency (NT) scan This may be offered during your dating scan or between 11 and 14 weeks. It measures the fluid under the skin at the back of your baby's neck. Many Down's syndrome babies have an increased amount of fluid in this area.

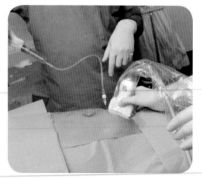

Amniocentesis This involves inserting a needle into your womb, and removing amniotic fluid for testing. Normally done after 14 weeks, it checks for abnormalities such as Down's syndrome. Preliminary results may be available in 48 hours.

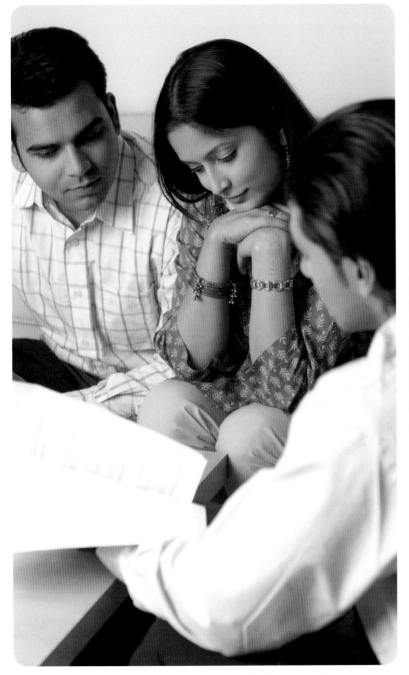

The results Your doctor or midwife will explain the results of your screening tests to you, and offer guidance if there is anything unexpected. In some cases, you may wish to have further diagnostic tests to clarify preliminary results, although this is never mandatory.

Interpreting the results

Your doctor or midwife will fully explain the implications of your test results to you, so that you can make any necessary decisions.

★ Rhesus factor: if you have a negative blood type and your baby is Rhesus-positive, your body could produce antibodies that could in future pregnancies destroy blood cells in your baby's circulation, so you will need an Anti-D injection.

★ HIV/AIDS: if you do have the infection (or carry it), steps can be taken to reduce the chances of it being transmitted to your baby.

★ Haemoglobin: if your red blood cell count is lower than 11, you may be anaemic and will need to increase your intake of iron (see p.25).

★ Hepatitis B: if you have this, your baby can be given a vaccine and antibodies to protect his liver.

★ Rubella: if your test shows that you are not immune, you should inform your doctor if you have been in contact with the disease.

★ STDs: if you test positive for conditions such as syphilis or chlamydia, you will have a variety of treatment options such as antibiotics.

★ NT test: an NT measurement of up to 2mm is normal at about 11 weeks, and up to 2.8mm by 13 weeks. A higher figure may not necessarily mean a problem, so you may wish to have CVS (see opposite) or amniocentesis, too.

★ CVS: results will indicate if there are chromosomal abnormalities, but you may wish to have amniocentesis to double check.

★ Amniocentesis: these results will indicate whether your baby is clear of chromosomal abnormalities.

High risk pregnancies

Some women are at greater risk of complications than others when they are pregnant, and will need specialist care throughout the antenatal period. If you fall into this category, try not to be alarmed. Calmly following the advice of your doctor and midwife will give you every chance of having a healthy baby.

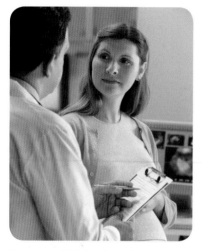

Are you at risk? Conditions that can cause complications include high blood pressure, heart disease, diabetes, kidney and auto-immune disorders, and cancer. Good antenatal care will help to detect and treat them.

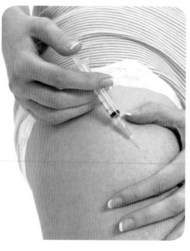

Gestational diabetes This occurs when pregnancy hormones block the usual action of insulin. You'll be given dietary guidelines to follow and, if this doesn't manage insulin levels, you may need injections or tablets.

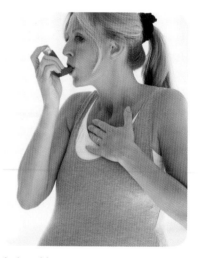

Asthma Many women experience changes in their asthma. Continuing with your medication can help to prevent an attack that might deprive your baby of oxygen, but you may need to change your dosage.

Other problems

There are several other conditions that may be either pre-existing or that may develop, which can potentially affect your pregnancy and the health of your baby. These include:

Being overweight This increases the likelihood of complications (such as pre-eclampsia, gestational diabetes, post-partum haemorrhage, thrombosis and urinary tract infections). It can also make procedures such as scanning and palpation more difficult. While pregnancy is no time to diet, eating well should help to balance your weight.

Being underweight There is an increased risk of miscarriage if you are very underweight; and if your diet is poor or inadequate, your baby's growth will be affected, she is at higher risk of birth defects, and also more likely to be born prematurely. It is possible to increase your weight by adopting a healthy diet, with the help of a dietician.

High risk factors In general, a pregnancy may also be considered higher risk if you:
★ Are older than 35, or younger than 15.
★ Are pregnant with more than one baby.
★ Have gestational diabetes (see above).
★ Have bleeding or threatened miscarriage.
★ Have had a premature baby in the past.
★ Have had a baby with a birth defect.

Miscarriage

Miscarriage occurs in three out of every 10 pregnancies and can be a devastating experience, although many women who suffer them go on to have successful pregnancies in the future.

Symptoms These can include vaginal bleeding (anything from light spotting to heavy bleeding, which may contain blood clots, brown discharge, and tissue), cramping and pain in your pelvis and back, and a cessation of pregnancy symptoms, such as nausea. Sometimes there are no symptoms, and your miscarriage is discovered during a routine scan.

Causes Most miscarriages occur in the first 12 weeks of pregnancy and more than half of all early ones are the result of a problem with genetic material that occurred when the egg and sperm came together. Other causes are hormone imbalances, immune problems, and infections, such as listeria. Miscarriage is more likely to occur in older mums, because egg quality declines with age. Smoking, alcohol consumption, multiple pregnancies, and possibly even stress are all known to be potential causes, too.

Treatment If your miscarriage is complete (your womb is empty and your cervix has closed), you won't need treatment, although you will need support. An incomplete miscarriage means that there is still pregnancy tissue in your womb, which will have to be removed, usually with medication to encourage your body to expel the contents of the womb, or by surgery.

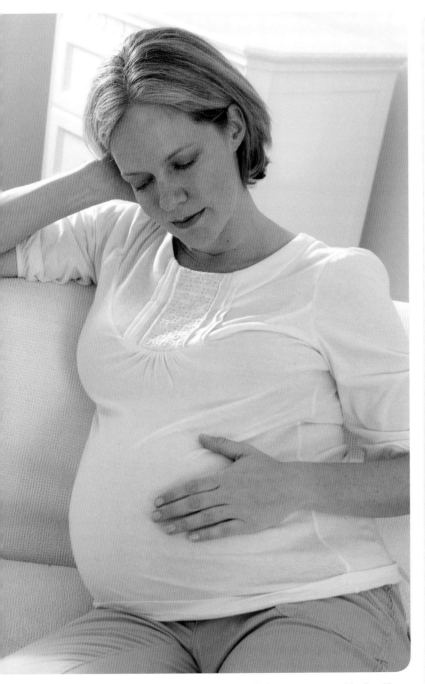

Age Although most older mums have no difficulties at all, they are at greater risk of problems with the placenta, miscarriage, and having babies with birth defects. And because things such as high blood pressure tend to develop with age, older mums may be in the high risk category.

Bonding with your bump

Although in the early days you may be preoccupied with symptoms such as nausea and fatigue, as your baby grows and begins to move you may find that you develop a warm, nurturing relationship well before he is even born.

Stimulating your baby

As early as the eighth week of pregnancy, the nerve endings that perceive touch have appeared on your baby's skin, and by the 10th week his brain's neurons have begun to form connections in response to repeated sensory experiences.

★ Spend time getting to know your baby. He can be stimulated in all sorts of ways when he is awake (see opposite).

★ Play some loud music, which not only wakes your baby but may stimulate him to move – and possibly even to the beat!

★ Lie down on your side with your bump supported; this seems to stimulate your baby to move to accommodate this new position.

★ A sweet, icy-cold drink may nudge him into action.

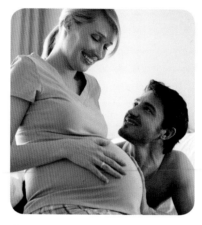

Your partner He can begin to establish the relationship that will last a lifetime. Your baby will recognize familiar voices when he is born, so encourage your partner to chat.

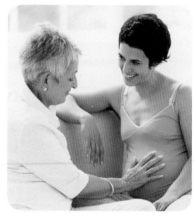

Touch The excitement of a new baby can be infectious, and friends and family will love the chance to feel your baby's ever-increasing movements.

KEY FACT

Studies have shown that by the 24th week, your baby's heart rate increases in response to you stroking or patting your abdomen.

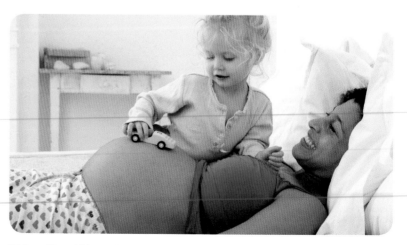

Siblings Your children will be bemused by the concept of a baby growing in mummy's tummy, and if they are encouraged to "meet" and talk to their new brother or sister early on, they'll find the process of adjusting to the prospect of a new arrival much easier.

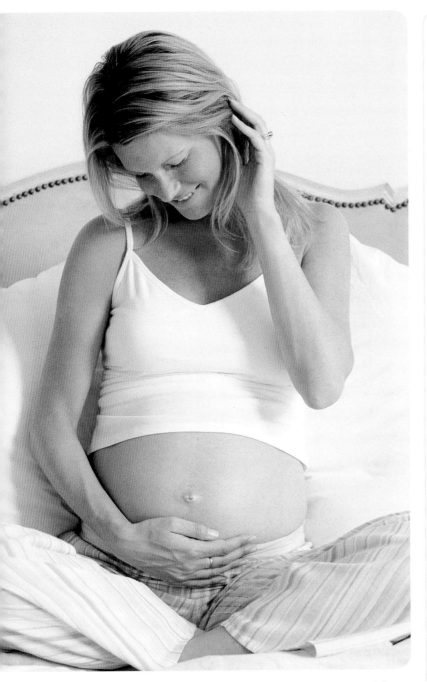

Take time to get to know your baby If you are busy and on the go all day, your baby will be lulled to sleep by the regular movement. He'll often wake up when you are relaxed and still. Sit quietly and you'll find that he responds to your voice and touch.

How will your baby respond?

Your baby will be aware of you from very early on in pregnancy, and once you feel those first flutterings, you can begin to play.

Noises As your baby grows and develops, he will increasingly respond to your stimulation. By the fifth month, his hearing is well developed, and he will respond to music and voices. He'll be most familiar with your voice, but he'll hear anyone who gets close. Don't forget that with all the blood rushing around your body, your heart beating, along with everything else, it's noisy in there!

Play games Push his foot or elbow when he moves it, and watch him respond. If you do it over and over again, he'll recognize it as being familiar. You've just had your first fun together. It's never too early to begin reading to your baby, either; most children's books have a rhythm that will soothe, and help him to understand the nuances of language.

Sing the same song Keep singing the same song to him; when he emerges, you may be able to use it comfort him.

Your baby's eyes At around 27 weeks, these will open, and he will respond to light. Get your bump out into the sunlight from time to time, or even shine a torch on it.

Twins If you are expecting twins, your babies will already have a close relationship and may move about in the womb (perhaps patting or pushing against each other) in a rather bumpy, haphazard way.

Your baby's first movements

Many women report first feeling their baby's movements around the fourth month of pregnancy, although second-time mums may recognize them much earlier. Whichever the case, feeling those flutterings is a magical experience, and offers your first real proof that your baby is "alive and kicking".

What is your baby doing?

Long before you feel her movements, your baby will be performing ever-more sophisticated actions as the weeks go by.

Early days Your baby will be wriggling and turning as she explores her new environment.

Nine weeks From around this time, your baby will hiccup, and will be able to move her arms and legs on her own. You won't feel these movements yet, but you'll soon know when she's got the hiccups – rhythmic little jerks are the sign to look for.

10 weeks Your baby will be able to bring her hands up and even yawn. Only as she gets a little bigger will you feel thumps against the inside of your abdomen as she kicks.

15–20 weeks You can expect to feel the first flutters by now, and it will feel much like having a goldfish flipping around inside you. These tiny movements are known as "quickening".

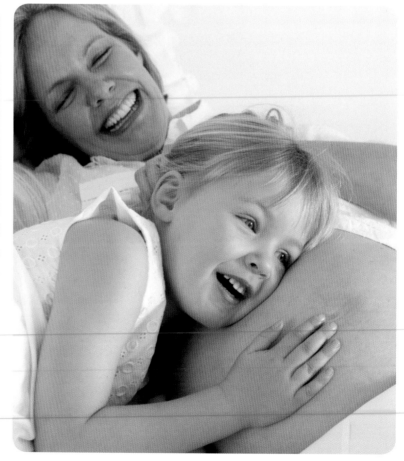

Sibling bonding Your little ones will enjoy feeling their new sibling-to-be kicking and squirming. Encourage them to get up close and begin the bonding process early. They will be surprised and delighted to receive a little kick or even feel shudders if your baby hiccups.

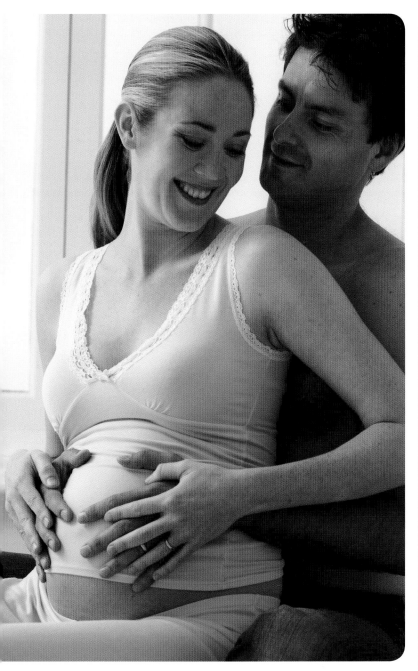

Dad-to-be For the first time your partner will be able to really share your pregnancy experience as he feels his new baby making her presence known. Many babies are more active in the evenings or when you are trying to sleep (a sign of things to come), so snuggle up close with your partner and let him enjoy his first hands-on contact with his child.

New movements

It won't be long before you'll be able to recognize what your baby is up to, and feel very specific sensations as she kicks, somersaults, turns, and makes herself comfortable.

Developing baby As she becomes a little older, you can expect an increase in activity, and don't be surprised if much of this occurs at night. Your movements during the day will literally rock or lull her to sleep, so when you relax, she may wake up. You may even feel something similar to somersaults, and that's exactly what she's doing.

32 weeks At around this time your baby's activities will peak, and you'll be able to feel definite movements as she becomes more cramped in her uterine home. You may be able to see your abdomen move as her little knees, head, elbows, and feet shift around as she changes her position.

36 weeks Your baby may shift into a head-down position around now, and you will feel stabs and wallops into your ribcage as she negotiates her space. It may be uncomfortable! As your baby gets larger, she will not be quite as active, and you may experience her movements as slow stretches rather than vigorous kicks and punches. She doesn't have much room by 36 weeks, so she'll be making the most of it. You'll notice that your baby is quiet when she sleeps, and much more vigorous when awake.

40 weeks You should still feel your baby moving regularly, although the movements may be smaller. If you experience fewer than 10 in a 12 hour day then contact your midwife.

More than one

Discovering that you are pregnant with more than one baby can be a shock, and you may need time to get used to the idea. Being a higher-risk pregnancy, you can expect a higher level of antenatal care, but many women sail through.

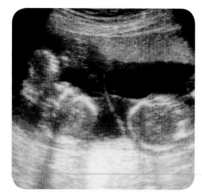

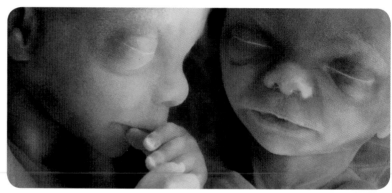

Dating scan You may not know you are carrying twins or triplets until your scan at 10 to 14 weeks. If there are twins in your family you are more likely to have them yourself.

Will they be identical? There are two types of twins: fraternal and identical. Identical twins are less common than fraternal because they result from the splitting of a single fertilized egg. Fraternal twins occur when two separate eggs are fertilized by two separate sperm and implant in the womb at the same time.

Twins in the womb

If you are expecting identical twins, who are created from the same set of genes, you may be surprised to find that they can be quite different sizes. This anomaly occurs because some twins share a placenta, and sometimes one will get more nutrition than the other.

Identical twins There are three ways that identical twins can develop and be carried:
★ One placenta feeds both babies. There can, however, be two amniotic sacs. This is referred to as having a "mono-chorial" placenta and "bi-amniotic".
★ One placenta and one amniotic sac shared by both babies is called "mono-chorial" placenta and "mono-amniotic".
★ Two placentas and each baby has its own amniotic sac. This is a "bi-chorial" pregnancy that is "bi-amniotic".

Fraternal twins These are two separate pregnancies that just happened to occur at the same time. Each baby has his own amniotic sac and placenta, so this is a "bi-chorial" and "bi-amniotic" pregnancy.

Twin-to-twin transfusion syndrome
This occurs when identical twins share a placenta and one receives less than normal quantities of blood, while the other receives too much. This is a potentially dangerous condition but there are treatments available.

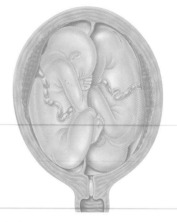

Positions Here one baby has his head down and the other is in the breech position. Your babies will simply make the best use of the available space.

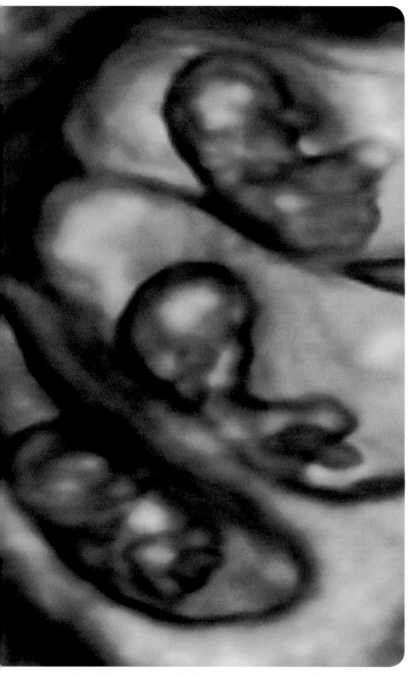

Carrying triplets This can create a significant physical and emotional strain; you will need to reduce your daily exercise, and have more scans, antenatal appointments, and tests to check that your babies are developing properly. Try to take things slowly and nurture yourself.

Twin pregnancy

Carrying twins or triplets puts you in the "higher-risk" category. You should receive extra care, but there are also things you can do to help make your pregnancy easier.

Eat more In total you should consume about 2,700 calories a day, based on a fresh, whole food diet.

Extra work You'll be more tired than a mum carrying a single baby – not only will there be extra weight (see p.45), but your own body will be nourishing two (or more) human beings, probably with an extra placenta and extra amniotic fluid. Backache is common, as is increased blood pressure. Take time to rest and put your feet up to avoid swelling. You may need to consider stopping work sooner, and factor in a pre-term birth. Many multiples are born early by Caesarean section, to prevent the complications that might accompany a natural birth.

Get support It will take time to come to terms with the idea of being parents to two babies at once; talk to other parents of twins, work out the practicalities (including expenses), and borrow whatever equipment you can.

Be prepared Twins are more likely to need some time in special care after the birth, so if you have other children you may need to make arrangements for their care.

Breastfeeding is possible You can breastfeed twins; get some advice from a breastfeeding counsellor before they are born to maximize your chances of success. Don't worry, you will make enough milk to feed two.

Antenatal classes

Antenatal classes are an excellent way to meet other prospective parents and form a support network that can be extended long after the birth. You'll also learn what to expect during labour, as well as the best methods for coping with pain and discomfort before and after the birth.

Choosing a class

There is a huge range of classes available, with many being run by the NHS. Your choice will be dictated by the area in which you live and, perhaps, your finances, but you may want to consider the following:

★ Try to find a class where the women have roughly the same due dates, which helps to establish bonds that will last after the birth.

★ If you don't have time for a full course, which normally runs for five to six weeks, you can consider one-day or half-day workshops.

★ You may find it helpful to go to more than one type of class.

★ Make sure the class allows lots of time for questions and discussion.

★ Make sure your class offers advice on how to cope with labour pain and the opportunity to experiment with different birth positions.

★ It's very helpful to have some guidance on how to cope after your baby is born, and the types of things that might go wrong.

★ You should feel comfortable in whatever class you choose.

★ Choose a class that works with your schedule. Although you are legally able to take time off work to attend them, your partner may not be able to manage daytime classes.

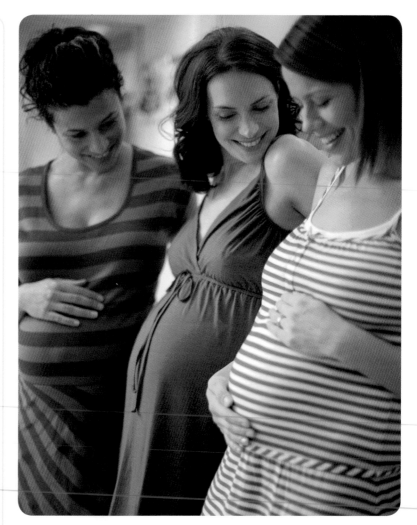

A ready-made set of friends The friendships made in antenatal classes can last for years. Your babies will be the same age, and you will be going through the same things at the same time, so you will be well positioned to swap tips and empathize with each other.

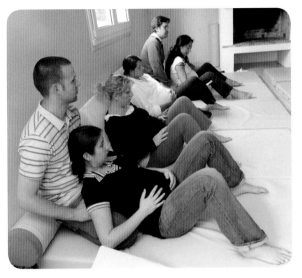

Your partner Make sure that he is involved in your antenatal classes; he'll need to know what to expect when the big day comes, and may find it reassuring to see other dads in the same position. A good class will offer plenty of advice for birth partners.

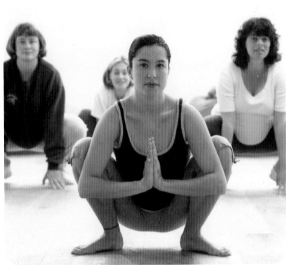

Active birth classes Also called yoga birth, these use exercise and yoga to strengthen your body in advance of the birth; you'll be taught breathing and relaxation as well as ways to improve your posture and circulation. These can complement your "couples" class well.

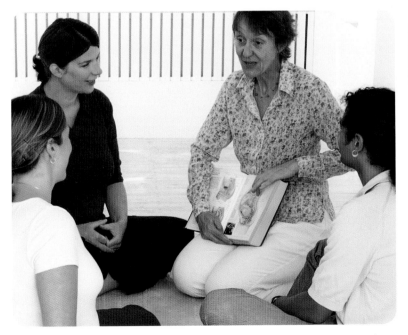

Types of classes Private classes are usually smaller, and encourage friendship among members; they normally incur a charge. NHS classes are usually held in a health centre or hospital, and are run by health professionals. Groups tend to be quite large, but the classes are free.

Which class?

The National Childbirth Trust runs the widest network of private classes but you may also wish to consider:

★ Early-pregnancy classes – these are designed for women who would like some guidance in the first months, with help and advice on nutrition, exercise, screening tests, symptoms, and emotional changes.
★ Refresher classes – these are aimed at women (or parents) who already have children, and offer an opportunity to find out the latest advice and research.
★ Consider carefully the organization running the course that you choose. Make sure it offers plenty of information on all forms of pain relief, and that it clearly explains why and when any intervention might be necessary.

Planning for the birth

Although it may be months until your baby's due date, it makes sense to investigate your options. Talk to your midwife and your partner about the type of birth you'd like to have and draw up a birth plan detailing the ideas you'd like to be considered.

Your birth plan choices

You can add anything to your birth plan to make the experience as positive as possible for you, your partner, and your baby. You might like to consider:

★ Your birthing environment: dim lights, music, a birthing ball to use for pelvic rocking, a beanbag, a private room, and what you'd like to wear.

★ Induction or acceleration of labour.

★ Who you'd like with you during labour.

★ How active you'd like to be – walking, doing some Pilates or yoga, using a birthing pool.

★ How you want your baby's heartbeat to be monitored.

★ Your pain relief choices.

★ What intervention is acceptable to you, and under what circumstances (remember however, that a medical emergency would require the decision to be taken by the doctor in charge).

★ The position in which you'd prefer to give birth to your baby.

★ An episiotomy if it is advised.

★ Having your baby placed directly on your chest before being cleaned.

★ What you want to do with the placenta when it has been delivered.

★ Your ideal hospital stay.

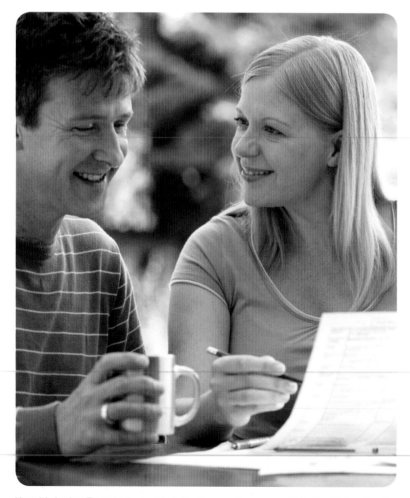

Your birth plan Try not to be too idealistic when you draw up your birth plan. Make a list of priorities with your partner. Remember that everything might not go according to plan in the labour room, so try to be flexible, and make sure you are both comfortable with your choices.

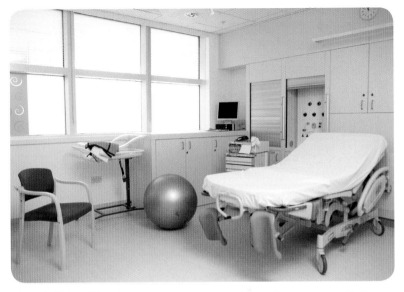

A hospital birth This makes sense for many women, because it means that medical care and the necessary equipment is on hand in the case of an emergency. Other women prefer the comfort of their own homes, and aim to have as little intervention as possible. Ask your midwife about what might be possible for you in your area and circumstances.

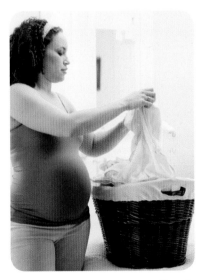

A home birth Women with uncomplicated pregnancies are often keen on a home birth, and there is good evidence that it can lead to a more positive, faster labour. You'll need to make arrangements for this well in advance, as well as making preparations of your own.

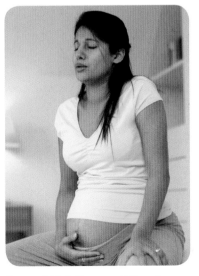

A natural birth If you would like to have as natural a birth as possible, it's important to practise some techniques such as breathing and positive visualization. They are usually taught in antenatal classes, and your partner will need to learn how to help you with them.

Creating a birth plan

Your birth plan provides you with an opportunity to focus on the different aspects of your care during labour and your baby's birth, and you can make it as detailed as you like.

Prepare to be flexible Bear in mind that you should only use your birth plan as a guide, and that circumstances can change significantly during the labour process. Remember that the most important thing is that you have a healthy baby at the end of it all.

Ask for guidance When you've put together your plan, show it to your midwife and ask her advice. She'll be happy to help you with any information you need, and point you in a different direction if parts of your plan are unrealistic for you.

Make copies Give your birth partner, your midwife, and the midwife attending your birth, a copy.

Natural remedies If you plan to employ a complementary therapist or use natural remedies, check this first with your midwife or the hospital. Make a note of what remedies you plan to use and when you will need them.

Highlight what is important You may need to change your mind, but if something is important to you, your carer should know about it.

Make a list It's helpful to note down things you would consider in every circumstance, giving your carers some options.

Getting organized

It's amazing how quickly nine months can pass, and you may suddenly find that you have entered the first stage of labour without any of your plans in place. The earlier you begin to get organized, the easier it will all be.

Things to do before the birth

★ **Get your hospital bag packed.** Having that ready will prevent you having the task hanging over your head and scrabbling around at the last minute.

★ **Make a list** of everyone you'd like contacted after the birth.

★ **Sort your baby's new clothes** into sizes, so you don't have to rummage around to find something that fits.

★ **Prepare your birth announcements** – address and stamp envelopes, or design something that can be sent via the internet, slotting in your new baby's photo and details once she's here.

★ **Get your finances in order** – pay outstanding bills, and budget for the coming months. You won't want to deal with reminders when you have your arms full with your new baby.

★ **Organize your work** so that your replacement can step in with ease.

TOP TIP

Why not produce something creative? Start a scrapbook, or simply write a letter to your baby to put in a keepsake box.

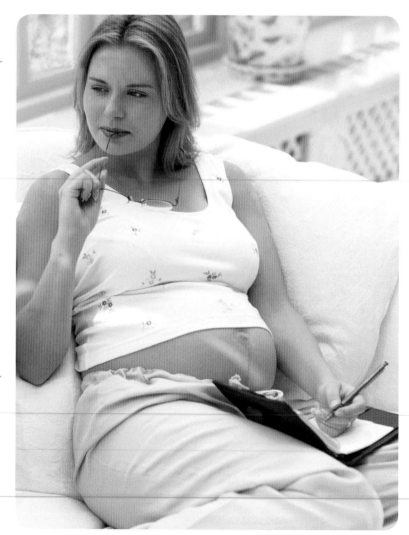

Keep a book of lists Use a page for each element that needs to be prepared. Consider everything from finances, maternity leave, and your baby's clothing and equipment, to your birth plan, your hospital bag, and even the shopping. Try to cross a few things off each day.

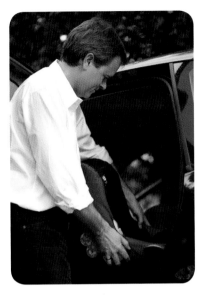

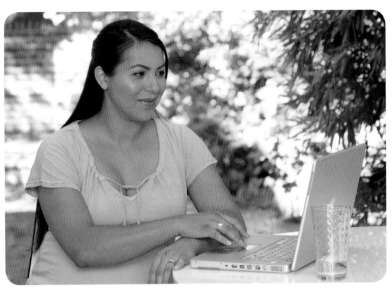

Buy the essentials Babies don't need a lot of equipment, but it's important that you get the basics, such as her cot, car seat, and pushchair, organized in advance. Give them all a trial run so you know how to use them.

Online shopping Order your groceries in advance on the internet and arrange to have everything delivered to your home. You can create and save a number of lists, and then just use them as required. You may also want to investigate what else may be available from your supermarket; it's helpful to know if you can get breastpads, nappies, barrier creams, and baby bath at the same time that your weekly grocery order arrives.

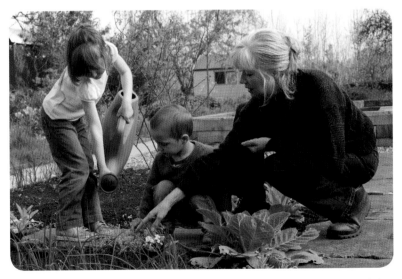

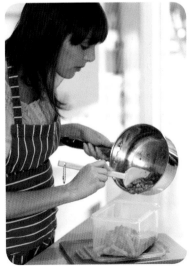

Planning childcare A new baby can be disorientating for your other children, particularly if you will be disappearing off to the hospital for a day or so. Make sure you have your plans in place well in advance, and that your little ones understand what's going to happen. Why not arrange a few trial runs with your parents or a good friend that they already know, so that they have something familiar and comforting to look forward to.

Batch cooking This is a must in the weeks leading up to the birth. Try to make an extra portion or two when you are cooking your main meals, and freeze them. They will be invaluable standbys when things get busy.

Your hospital bag

No baby arrives to a set schedule – so having your hospital bag packed will help make sure that you are ready when your baby is! Even if you are expecting to have a home birth, it's worth putting together a bag just in case things don't go according to plan.

Don't forget

Check what your hospital recommends you take; you may also find that they provide some of the things you had planned to pack. Remember to bring:

★ A little extra of everything, just in case your stay is longer than anticipated.

★ Items that will make your environment more personal, such as pillows and towels.

★ Any regular medication you are taking (check with your doctor if you are planning to breastfeed).

★ Pain relief, such as your TENS machine and any homoeopathic remedies (see pp.94 & 112).

★ Your baby's hospital bag, including nappies and toiletries (see pp.74–75).

★ Relaxation materials: books, magazines, and even an iPOD or portable CD player can help to while the hours away; soothing or upbeat music may also get you in the right frame of mind.

★ Comfortable going-home clothes: you won't be ready to return to your pre-pregnancy ones just yet.

★ Your baby's car seat – it's amazing how many people forget that the car seat will be absolutely necessary to get your new arrival home.

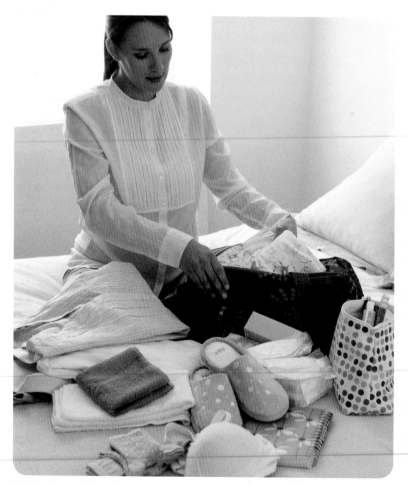

Being prepared Even if you are hoping for a quick stay, your hospital bag will ideally contain everything that you and your baby might need for a few days in hospital. You'll also need to put together anything you may need during the labour itself. Try to involve your birth partner in the process, so he knows what you have packed – and why.

TOP TIP

Most parents-to-be get to hospital in plenty of time, but when your contractions begin, call your midwife to let her know what's going on.

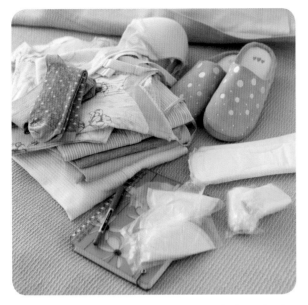

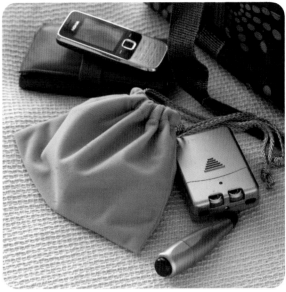

Items for labour and afterwards Bring your birth plan, a dressing gown, slippers, a nightie or old T-shirt for labour, and spare pyjamas or nightie for after the birth. Old or disposable knickers and sanitary towels will be essential after your baby is born and don't forget your nursing bra and some breastpads.

Mobile phone, purse, and TENS machine Don't forget to pack your TENS machine (see p.94). Your birth experience may take some time and you may have an unexpected stay in hospital. Money for extras, an iPOD or portable CD player, and your mobile phone are useful items, no matter what type of labour you have planned.

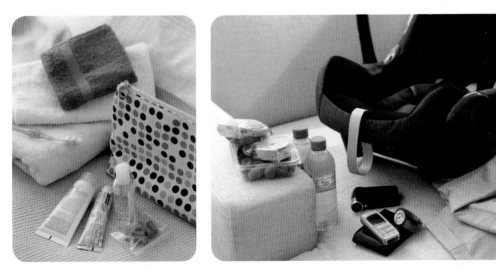

Toiletries Remember to bring a toothbrush and toothpaste, a clean towel, and flannel. Shampoo, soap, and shower gel will refresh you after the labour. Nipple cream and some earplugs can also be useful.

Your birth partner's bag Put him in charge of snacks and drinks (to keep your blood-sugar level stable and your energy levels high), as well as the carseat, camera, money, telephone, a watch to time contractions, and another copy of your birthplan. He may also wish to bring some toiletries and a change of clothing. It's a good idea, too, to bring things to provide distraction in the quieter moments, such as board games or a deck of cards.

Your baby's hospital bag

You'll be amazed by how many things your new baby will need on her arrival, and how quickly she'll go through nappies and clothing. Ask your midwife for an idea of her expected weight, so that you can buy the appropriate size.

TOP TIP

Ask your hospital what they supply; some will provide nappies, toiletries, and blankets. Some birth centres may prefer you to use cloth nappies rather than disposables.

What she will need

★ A "layette" set will provide the basic clothing that your baby will need. A couple of these, along with some nappies, toiletries, and blankets, will see her through the first few days.

★ Buying an all-white layette may sound boring, but it is actually much easier to keep it clean. You can treat stains on white fabrics easily, and often with natural products.

★ Go "disposable" whenever you can; disposable nappies, bibs, and even changing mats can be a bonus, to clear away the mess completely with the minimum of fuss. It will also save you from creating a mountain of laundry, too.

★ Choose cotton, machine-washable clothing. Natural fabrics "breathe" and can help to prevent overheating. They are also gentle on your baby's new skin.

★ Choose specifically designed (preferably fragrance-free) baby products and use sparingly – her skin will be very sensitive.

★ Consider washing her clothes and towels before you pack them in her bag – they'll be softer without their "finish", and they won't have any chemicals that can irritate your baby's skin.

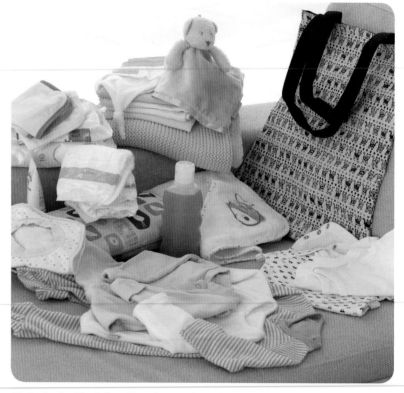

All the basics Your baby will need: 1–2 nighties (for boys, too), 2–3 babygros, 2–3 cotton vests, 1–2 cotton bibs, 3–4 muslin squares, a cardigan and soft hat (in the event that it gets cool, or you wish to take her on a stroll around the hospital grounds); a folding changing mat, nappies, toiletries, and baby wipes; a hooded towel and flannel; and a soft receiving blanket or shawl for your new arrival. It's also a great idea to introduce her to a soft toy or comfortable blanket which she will find familiar and soothing later on.

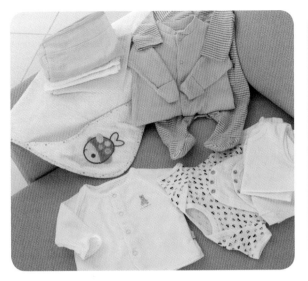

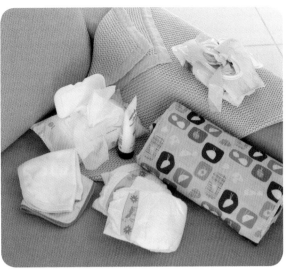

Pack the right clothes for the hospital Baby nighties are ideal for easy access to your baby's nappy, and can allow quick changes when she's fractious or sleeping. Choose babygros and vests with poppers, as zips and buttons can be uncomfortable. Although hospitals are usually hot, your baby will need a cardigan and hat if the temperature drops. Muslins and bibs will protect her clothing (and yours) from milk and other leaks and spills.

A mini changing station Create one in your baby's bag, with everything you need to get her cleaned up. You'll need at least 12–24 disposable nappies; newborn sizes will usually fit most babies, but check to see if your midwife thinks you are carrying a bigger baby. Bring a travel changing mat, some cotton wool, a pack of disposable, fragrance-free water-based wipes, as well as some gentle baby bath and some nappy sacks to dispose of used nappies.

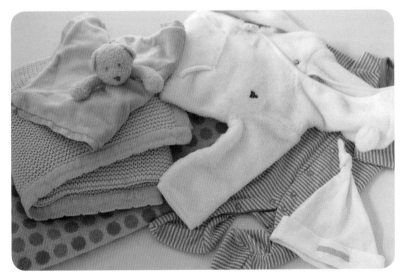

Going home Choose something that is comfortable and easy to remove, for going home. Bring a light blanket to keep her warm, her "comfort" toy or blanket, and, her car seat. When outside, all young babies should wear hats for the first few weeks, to help them maintain their body temperature, but make sure that she isn't too hot once inside the car.

Expect the unexpected

Always pack more than you think you may need for your hospital stay. Complications can mean that you are there for longer than expected.

Be prepared Babies can also be unbelievably messy. Nappy explosions and leaks are very common, and your baby will also take some time to catch on to the art of feeding, and dribble and posset up a good proportion of her milk, so choose easy-to-wash, comfortable clothing for you both, and bring plenty of disposable nappies and water-based wipes to the hospital.

Preparing for baby's arrival

It's helpful to get your home organized and well-stocked with essential supplies in advance of your baby's birth because spare time is going to be at a premium for quite a few weeks to come.

Baby safety

Once your baby is born, it will be only months before he can move, so you should consider the following:

★ Get into the habit of having hot drinks only in the kitchen; it's very easy to scald your baby with even minor spills.

★ Put a carpet or rug at the base of the changing table to cushion any falls.

★ Tape down rugs – you don't want to trip with a baby in your arms.

★ Make sure there are no strings, electrical sockets, cords, or anything that could pose a risk of strangulation or choking near to your baby's cot.

★ Consider getting a fire guard if your fireplace is regularly in use.

★ Keep small coins and sharp objects out of your baby's reach.

★ Place all medication, cleaning supplies, alcohol, laundry supplies, and toiletries in a child-proof cupboard that is preferably out of reach.

★ Secure bookshelves and chests of drawers to the wall – many babies become avid climbers very early on.

★ Install safety gates securely at the top and bottom of stairways.

★ Get down on your hands and knees to see exactly what could be a danger from your baby's perspective.

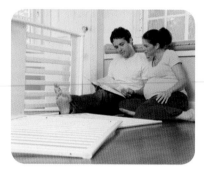

Assembling the cot Whether you have a full-sized cot for your baby or something smaller, such as a Moses basket or crib, make sure that you have it assembled, with the bedding in place, before you go into labour.

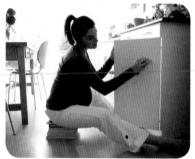

Nesting It's natural to find that you have an urge to clean just before your labour begins. Known as the "nesting" instinct, it will make your home more hygienic for your baby, and therefore help you to feel more relaxed.

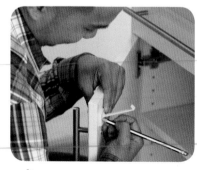

Baby-proofing Look carefully at the safety of your home. It may seem hard to believe, but your baby will be mobile in a few short months, and a house can be a potential source of accidents and injuries (see left).

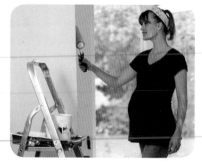

Decorating Choose low- or zero-VOC (volatile organic compound) paint, which does not contain the unhealthy chemicals found in traditional paints – now linked to a variety of health problems.

Useful gifts If you know that friends have baby showers or parties planned for you, you might want to consider asking them to club together to purchase some of the larger, more expensive items that will be required.

Baby essentials

Getting together everything your baby will need for the first few weeks and even months can take some time. Babies grow very quickly, so it's a good idea to save some money with borrowed clothing or hand-me-downs.

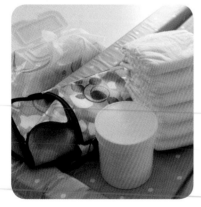

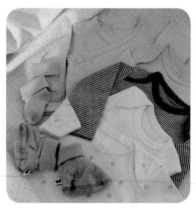

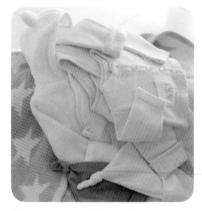

Outerwear Depending on the season and the climate where you live, you'll need some outerwear for your baby. Hats are essential in the early days, but choose something light so she doesn't overheat.

Vests Invest in at least half a dozen cotton, cross-over or envelope-necked vests with poppers at the crotch. In hot weather these make an ideal sleepsuit for naptimes. Some scratch mitts and socks are useful, too.

Sleepwear This should be cotton to prevent overheating. Layer blankets or use a baby sleeping bag that cannot be kicked off. Choose easy-to-fasten babygros – you may have to change her in the dark.

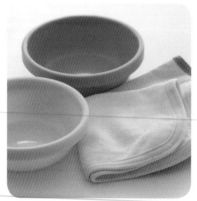

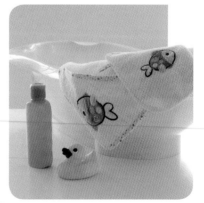

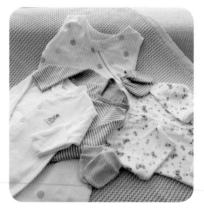

Nappy station You'll need a changing mat, baby wipes or a bowl for warm water, some cotton wool or a flannel, barrier cream, a good supply of nappies, and a place to dispose of them (see p.156–159).

Topping and tailing You will need two bowls, cotton wool or two boil-washed flannels. Remember to keep one bowl and flannel for cleaning her face only, and the others for the rest of her body (see p.161).

Bathtime Make sure your baby's bath is sturdy and easy to carry. A thermometer is useful to check the temperature (see pp.160–61) and you'll need gentle baby bath/shampoo and a hooded baby towel.

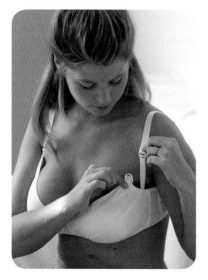

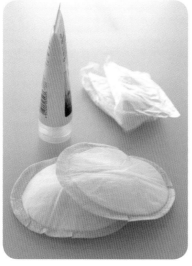

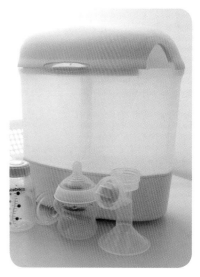

Nursing bras Have yourself measured for at least three comfortable nursing bras, which you'll need as soon as your baby is born. Make sure that you can open the fastenings easily – preferably with one hand.

Breastfeeding Prepare yourself for breastfeeding by buying breastpads to help absorb leaks and keep your breasts more comfortable, as well as a soothing lanolin or chamomile-based nipple cream.

Bottle-feeding If you plan to bottle-feed, you'll need bottles, teats, a sterilizer, and a bottle brush to keep things clean. If you plan to express your breastmilk you will also need this equipment as well as a pump.

Choosing nappies

You can choose between disposable or reusable nappies, and both have their pros and cons. It's worth remembering that whatever you choose, your baby will go through six to 10 nappies each day. Don't buy too many of the same size; new babies grow quickly.

Which nappies? Although disposables are undoubtedly convenient, reusable ones are becoming increasingly popular. Choose what suits you best, but as a compromise between the two, you could try using reusables during the day, and more absorbent disposables at night.

Reusable nappies:
★ Pins and fabric squares are no longer needed; now you can choose Velcro-closing nappies that are easily laundered.
Pros:
★ Your baby will be wearing soft, natural fibres next to her skin.
★ Apart from the initial outlay, these are cheaper in the long run.

★ Cloth ones produce less waste, and use fewer materials in their manufacture.
Cons:
★ Washing produces waste water, and uses cleansing agents and chemicals.
★ Washing can be time-consuming (if it's in your budget, you might want to consider a laundering service).
★ Changes will be more frequent, as reusables tend to be less absorbent.
★ They can take a long time to dry naturally or you may need to invest in a tumble dryer.
★ You will need accessories such as liners and plastic/rubber overpants.
★ You'll have to carry wet and soiled nappies home when you are out.

Disposable nappies:
Many are now biodegradable, made from natural products, and are chemical-free, but read the labels carefully.
Pros:
★ They are much more convenient, and do not require any additional accessories.
★ Fewer changes are necessary because they are super-absorbent and they cause fewer cases of nappy rash.
★ They fit better, causing fewer leaks.
Cons:
★ They are more expensive overall.
★ They produce high levels of waste.
★ They must be disposed of properly.
★ Some disposable nappies may contain man-made chemicals.

Your baby's bedroom

Planning and decorating your baby's nursery and buying his new equipment can be great fun; there are, however, several things to bear in mind. Safety must always be your first priority; remember, too, that babies grow quickly and some items may simply never end up being used.

Nursery basics

★ A cot, cradle, or Moses basket.

★ A changing table (make sure that it has a lip to prevent him from rolling off).

★ A changing mat – choose one that can be easily washed.

★ A baby monitor.

★ Basic toiletries (see p.78).

★ Newborn nappies (see p.79).

★ Toiletries and equipment for changing, topping and tailing (see p.78).

★ A mobile over the baby's cot.

★ A music box to play soothing tunes.

★ A soft rug or mat made of natural fibres, for tummy and playtime (tape it down, to prevent tripping).

★ A bouncy chair, that can be moved from room to room.

★ A night light.

★ A soft, dim light.

★ A comfortable chair for feeding or night-time settling.

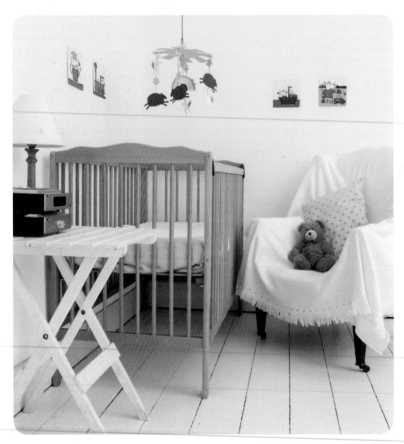

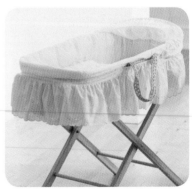

Choosing a cot Go for one with a drop-side as it will allow you to lift your baby without straining your back. If it has an adjustable height you should also be able to use it until he is ready to move to a bed. If your cot is second-hand, you must buy a new mattress. Look for one with an all-cotton filling or wool casings, and try to avoid those that contain the chemicals used in fire-retardant polybrominated diphenyl ethers (PBDEs).

Smaller cots Many babies sleep better in smaller confines when they are very young, so you may choose a Moses basket or cradle. These are, however, soon outgrown, so don't spend a fortune on one.

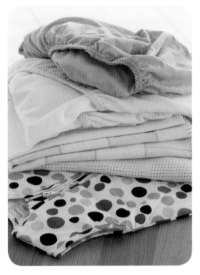

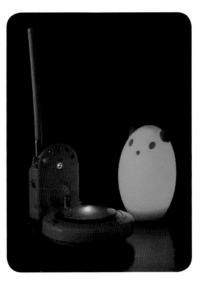

Cot essentials You'll need a mattress protector, fitted sheets for the mattress and a baby sleeping bag, or cotton sheets and light, cellular blankets for layering.

A baby monitor This is useful when your baby moves into his own room, but current advice is to keep your baby with you while he sleeps until he is six months old.

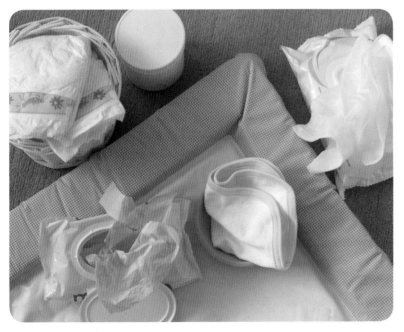

Changing station A changing table is not essential, and plastic changing mats can be used on almost any floor, so set up a few changing stations in other parts of the house for quick clean-ups and keep them stocked with the basics (see p.78).

Health and safety in your baby's room

Preparing your baby's nursery doesn't just involve decorating. You need to create a safe, nurturing environment in which he can grow and develop.

★ Duvets are not suitable for babies as they can be too warm and pose a risk of suffocation; layering cotton cellular blankets or using a baby sleeping bag can help to keep your baby at the right temperature.

★ Carpets can harbour dust mites, dirt, and allergens, and emit chemicals into the air; so if you can, choose hardwood floors paired with a rug made of all-natural fibres (such as wool, cotton, or hemp) and make sure that you vacuum twice a week.

★ If you can, choose all-wood furniture made with non-toxic finishes; furniture made from particle board or veneers can release harmful gases such as formaldehyde.

★ Bedding should be washable, and cotton; it should never contain flame-retardant PBDE (see opposite).

★ Make sure there are no strings, electrical sockets, electrical cords, or anything that could possibly pose a risk of strangulation or choking near to your baby.

★ Consider using a safety belt on your baby's changing table.

★ Do not put pillows, thick bedding, or any electrical items in the cot.

★ Make sure the mattress fits the cot snugly, so your baby can't slip between the mattress and frame.

★ Make sure all screws and bolts are secure, so that there is no danger of the cot collapsing, your baby being scratched by them, or choking.

Out and about

The day will soon come when you are ready to venture a little further afield with your baby, so take time now to research your options; good-quality slings, car seats, and pushchairs are expensive, but they will get plenty of use.

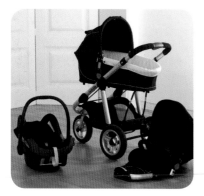

Travel systems These can include everything from carry cots and car seats to traditional pushchairs, all of which can be clipped to the same frame. Check carefully: a travel system may be cheaper than buying separate pieces of equipment.

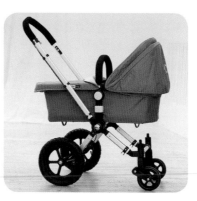

Traditional pram Although not essential, a pram will probably be more comfortable for your baby. It's useful, too, for impromptu naps inside the house, and if you have one that detaches from the base, you can also use it as a travel cot for the first few months.

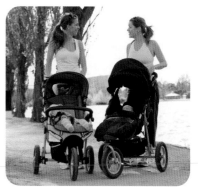

Being active Many mums enjoy jogging and walking with their babies strapped into a pushchair. If this is what you want to do, choose one with good suspension to keep your baby comfortable over bumps, and a high handle to prevent strain on your back.

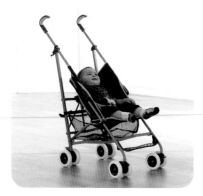

Foldable pushchairs Although convenient, most of these are not appropriate until your baby is at least six months old, because she needs more support until she can sit properly. Look for one with a fully reclining, sturdy back so that your baby can lie flat.

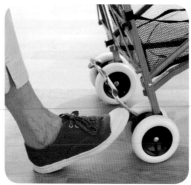

The brake This is a vital feature, and you need to know exactly how to use it. Ask for a demonstration, and practise using the brake before your baby arrives. Use it whenever you stop, as even the gentlest of inclines can lead to a runaway buggy.

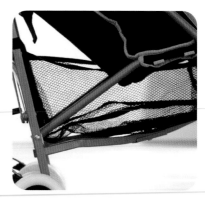

Storage space Choose a pushchair with adequate, inbuilt storage for your changing bag, toys, and, of course, your shopping. Although you can hang bags on the handles of your pushchair, it is unwise to do so as they can cause it to topple over backwards.

Sling and pushchair safety

By law, slings and pushchairs must be designed and manufactured in accordance with strict rules to ensure you baby's safety. Both items are essential equipment for all new parents, and are perfectly safe if you follow a few simple guidelines. Consider the following:

Sling safety It is recommended that you check that your baby's face is not covered, and is visible at all times. If you are breastfeeding your baby in a sling, change her position after her feed so that her head is facing up and is clear of both the sling and your body. It is very important that you check your baby frequently when she is in a sling. Soft carriers should carry the British Standards Institute (BSI) safety number: BS EN 13209 Part 2:2005. For the latest advice on the safety standards required for all baby equipment check the official website at: www.tradingstandards.gov.uk

A good fit Make sure that your sling fits properly and that it gives your baby adequate neck and back support. Your baby can easily fall out if it is too big for her and, if it is too small, there's a risk that she may overheat or even suffocate.

Pushchair safety All types should carry the BSI safety number: BS EN 1888:2003 and European safety standards number EN1888. Every pushchair should have a working brake and a five-point harness. Always fasten the harness, even on small babies, because if the pushchair should tip your baby could fall out.

Using pushchairs safely There should be two locking devices to hold your pushchair securely in place. Once the main lock has been released in order to collapse your pushchair, the secondary lock should be activated to stop it from collapsing. There should be no areas where your child's fingers could get caught in the collapsing mechanism. Check before you buy, and ask for a demonstration to make sure that you know exactly how to erect and collapse your pushchair safely. Choose a pushchair with a two-stage folding system, so that it will not collapse unexpectedly.

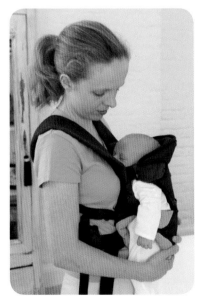

A soft carrier A great way to free your hands to get on with jobs around the house, a carrier allows you to transport your baby and keep her close to you. Make sure she has plenty of back support, and that her head doesn't fall forward.

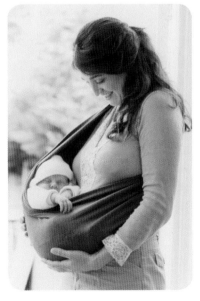

A sarong-style sling This keeps your baby in a natural position, and can allow easy breastfeeding when the moment arises. Take care, though: your baby must always be facing upwards, with her face clear of the sling fabric and you (see above).

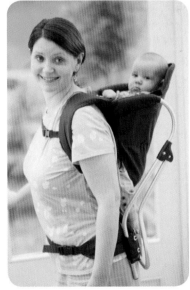

A backpack carrier These are suitable for older babies, who have more neck and back control. Choose one with wide straps so that you'll be comfortable as she becomes heavier. If more than one member of the family plans to use it, try it out first for size.

Choosing car seats

You'll need a car seat to take your baby home from hospital, so do some research in advance of his birth and make sure you buy one that fits your car. Choose one that is not only comfortable and safe for your baby, but which will provide him with the neck and head support he needs.

Choosing a car seat

Most car seats get a great deal of use, doubling up as a chair when you are out and about, and a snug resting place when your baby falls asleep in the car.

★ Make sure that your baby's car seat is light enough to carry, and has a sturdy, easy-to-manage handle.

★ Babies up to about 10kg (22lb) – or up to six to nine months – will need a rear-facing seat.

★ Some car seats are designed only for the first six or nine months; others can be adapted to face forward and carry babies up to about 13kg (29lb). These infant-toddler seats may last a little longer, but experts recommend choosing an infant seat first, as it is contoured to hold and protect your baby.

★ Make sure the harness is easy to fasten and unfasten; you will need to get him into the seat with minimum disruption and be able to release him quickly.

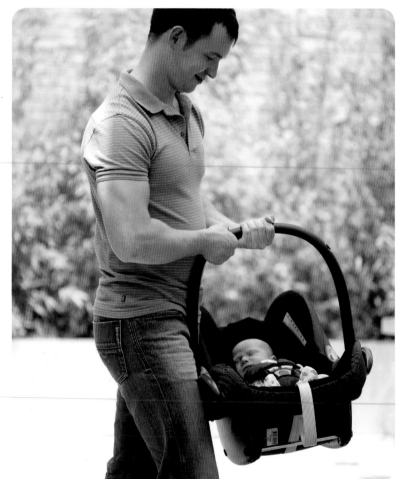

KEY FACT

No matter how upset your baby is, it is not safe to hold him on your lap in a car. In a crash he would be seriously injured, even if you are wearing a seatbelt.

Safely strapped in Your baby's seat should have a five-point harness that is easy to release, and sits firmly against his chest. Tighten the harness so that there is a finger-space of room between the strap and your baby. The straps should rest across the centre of his shoulders but make sure they aren't too tight, and that he is comfortable. A car seat that can be removed from the car with your baby still strapped in place is ideal if he falls asleep.

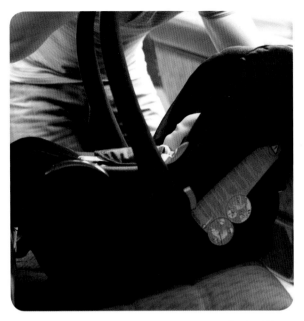

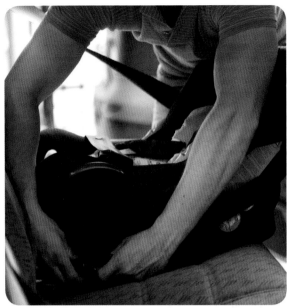

Rear-facing position Babies up to six to nine months should have rear-facing car seats, and be seated in the back seat of your car. If you have bucket seats, you may need to provide a wedge of Styrofoam or something similar to prevent the seat from rocking, and give it a firm base. Ask your car manufacturer for details.

Fasten the adult seatbelt The adult seatbelt should be stretched around the car seat, according to the manufacturer's instructions, taking care to weave the seatbelt through any fastenings on the seat itself. Ask for a thorough demonstration before you use the seat for the first time; it can be fiddly to experiment with your baby in situ.

Car seat safety

Your baby will spend a great deal of time in his car seat, so not only does it need to be comfortable, but safety is absolutely essential.

You should also check that it is compatible with your car. When buying your car seat, you should consider the following:

★ Always make sure that your car seat meets the latest safety standard, and has a British or European kitemark: ECE R44.03 or R44.04. Check the official website at www.tradingstandards.gov.uk

★ Experts recommend that you do not use a second-hand car seat.

★ Always fasten the harness properly, even if you are simply walking a short distance. It can be easy to forget, particularly if you cover your baby with a blanket before you leave your home.

★ Make sure that you place all blankets under your baby's arms while driving; if he shifts position, his blanket can ride up.

★ Don't tie anything to your baby's car seat, as it can cause accidental strangulation; only use accessories that are designed to fit the seat.

★ If you buy a car seat that's part of a travel system you can clip it directly into the pushchair or pram frame.

★ You may consider a car seat fitting service, to make sure that the seat you are planning to buy fits in your car. It's also important to check the length of your seatbelt, as some are not long enough to fit properly around the seat.

★ Make sure the buckle of your seat belt doesn't rest on the car seat; it can

damage it or break open in the event of an accident. Only the fabric part of the belt should touch the seat's frame.

★ Always make sure that your baby's car seat sits firmly in place, and won't shift when you apply pressure. Seats loosely fastened into place will provide your baby with little protection when you stop suddenly, or in the event of an accident.

★ A child restraint system called ISOFIX has points that are fixed connectors in a car's structure into which an ISOFIX child seat can simply be plugged. Check your car manufacturer's manual to be sure that the seat and car are compatible.

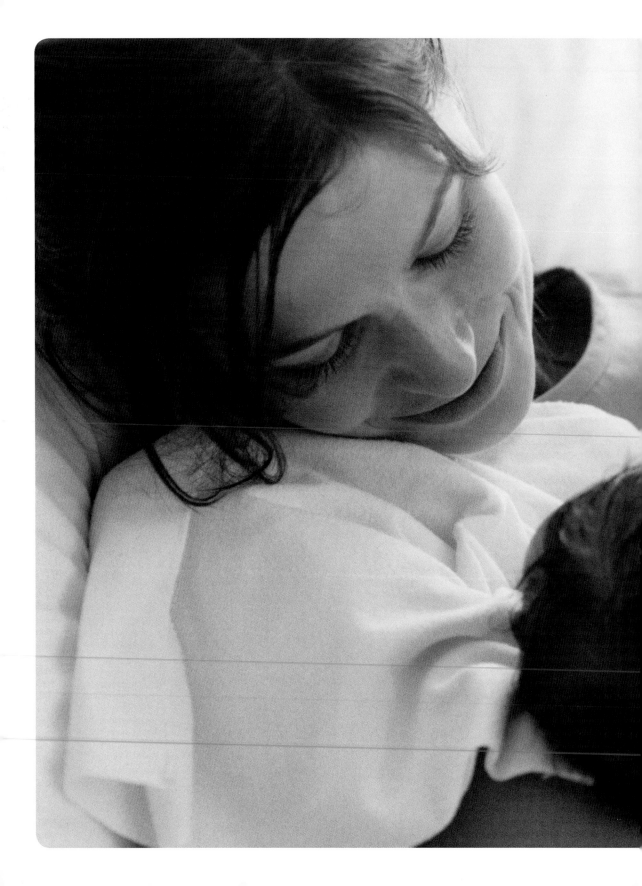

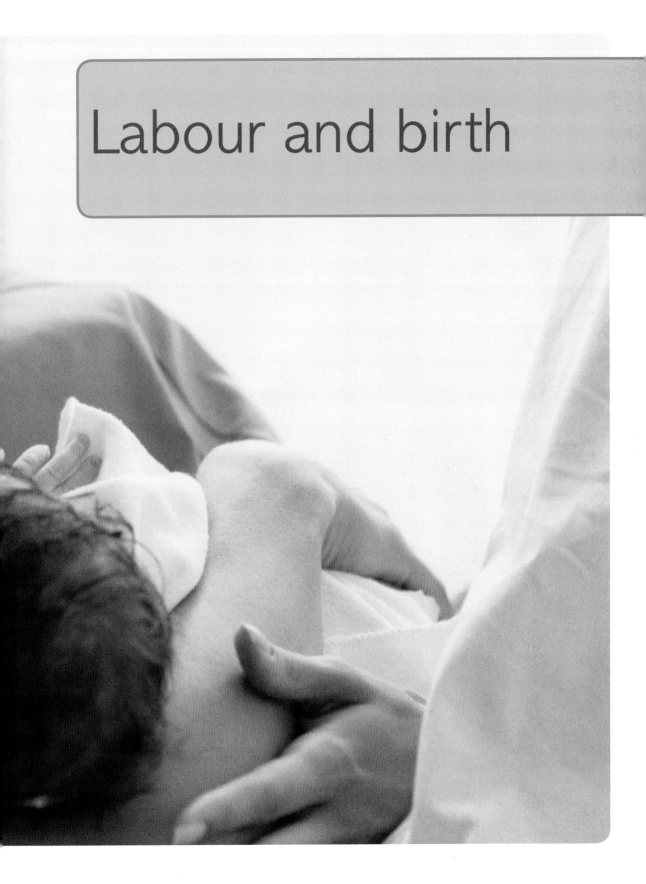

Labour and birth

GIVING BIRTH

Women have been giving birth since the advent of humanity, and it is a natural, positive process with a spectacular end result. Understanding the stages of labour, and the help that is available at each stage, can help you to feel confident and in control.

YOUR CHOICES

The most important thing to remember is that this birth is your moment, and you are perfectly entitled to create an experience that will be positive, productive and memorable for all the right reasons. This begins with the creation of your birth plan, which will outline everything that you'd like to experience as you give birth to your baby. You can choose where you have your baby, and you can create an environment that will be most conducive to the labour and delivery that you want.

UNDERSTANDING THE BASICS

Like pregnancy, childbirth is comprised of three stages, each of which has a defined role. Before you even enter the first stage, however, you may experience symptoms of "pre-labour", which can include practice contractions; "shows" – which is the discharge of the mucus plug that has sealed your cervix for the duration of your pregnancy; pressure on your lower half; an upset tummy; and something known as "lightening", which is when your baby drops down into your pelvis. Pre-labour can last for hours – or even weeks!

THE STAGES OF LABOUR

Once labour is established, you are officially in the first stage, when contractions become more frequent and intense as your baby moves deeper into your pelvis, and down through the birth canal. Contractions press your baby against your cervix, causing it to thin and dilate, and allow her to slip through. The duration of this stage varies widely between women, but it is usually the longest stage of labour. Staying active, positive, and relaxed can help to keep things moving, and reduce the discomfort involved. There are plenty of options for dealing with any discomfort and your midwife can help you make the choices that are right for you.

Just when you think you can't go on any longer – which is a sign of a mini-stage, known as "transition" – you'll enter the second stage of labour. Your cervix will now be fully dilated, and you will feel an urge to push. Your midwife will monitor this stage carefully, and help you to push with your natural instincts to bring your baby into the world. The second stage ends with the birth, then your baby's cord is cut and clamped, and you can begin the process of parenthood.

The final stage of your labour involves the delivery of the placenta, which has sustained your baby's life for many months while she was in your womb.

A LITTLE PRE-PLANNING

You can make many of the decisions about your labour well in advance of the big day, and for this reason it is important to ask questions and work out the pros and cons of all of the various options. Equally, however, it is crucial that you remain flexible and bear in mind that things don't always go to plan.

Focusing on the constructive things that you can do to make your labour as comfortable and positive as possible – such as learning breathing and relaxation techniques, using appropriate remedies or therapies, adopting positions that will encourage an easier delivery and keep things going, and making the best use of your midwife's skills and any pain relief on offer – will help to keep things on track. Before you know it, you'll have your beautiful new baby in your arms, and your life as a parent can finally begin.

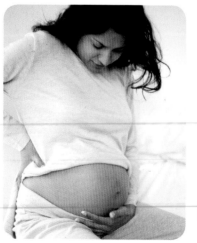

Managing the pain There are several pain relief options available, from breathing techniques through to a full epidural.

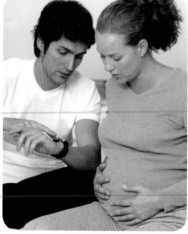

Timing contractions Ask your partner to help with timing how far apart your contractions are and how long they last.

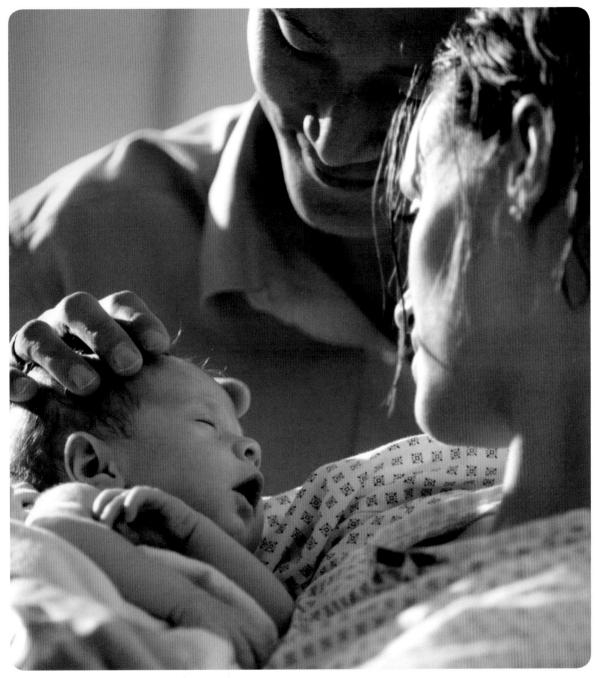

Welcome to the world At last, your labour and birth are over and your baby is in your arms. As the staff who have been involved give you some special time and space, you can enjoy the relative calm and savour the opportunity to greet and get to know your new baby. These first moments can seem overwhelming as you experience a huge range of emotions, ranging from relief and exhaustion to wonder and joy.

Your birth environment

The environment in which you have your baby is an important factor in making the birth a positive experience, and whether it takes place in hospital, at home, or at a birthing centre, you can help to make sure you have the birth that you want.

Your hospital visit

A tour of the hospital in which you plan to give birth is essential, as you'll be able to see first hand where you are likely to deliver your baby, and have an opportunity to ask questions.
You may want to know about:

★ Admissions procedures.

★ What you can – or can't – bring.

★ Intervention and Caesarean rates.

★ How the hospital treats birth plans.

★ What pain relief will be available, and if natural remedies are encouraged.

★ Fetal monitoring.

★ Who will be delivering your baby and how long the shifts are.

★ Whether there are birthing pools.

★ What happens after the birth and what support is on offer.

★ Whether your partner can stay over.

★ Visiting hours.

★ Parking and catering facilities.

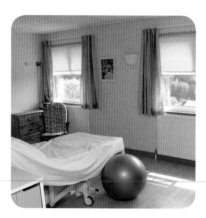

Hospital birth Many women feel more confident giving birth in hospital, where medical care is instantly available. You can usually choose your hospital, and normally book it at the start of your pregnancy.

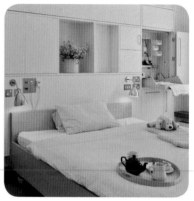

Birthing centres These offer personal attention and tend to focus on natural childbirth, but in the event of an emergency, such as a Caesarean being necessary, you should be prepared to transfer to a hospital.

KEY FACT
Many women now opt for an early six-hour discharge from hospital and go straight home from the delivery suite, so there's no need to be transferred to a postnatal ward.

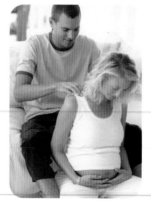

Your partner You need to make sure that your birth partner is well prepared, and understands exactly what he can do to help you.

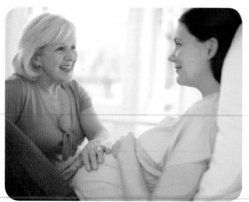

A close friend or relative Either of these may be a good, practical choice of birth partner if your baby's dad is likely to find the labour distressing. Remember that there's no reason why he can't come in a little later, to share your elation once your baby has arrived.

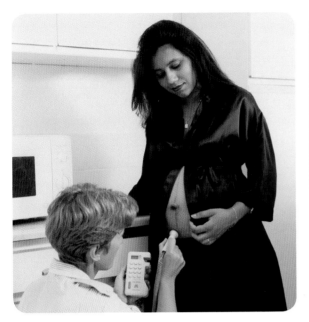

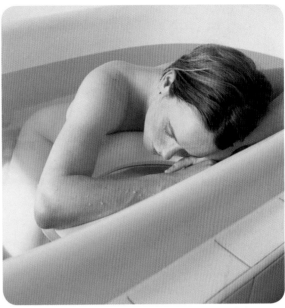

Home birth The healthcare policy in your area will determine whether you have a special home birth team who rotate their duties or a community midwife to care for you. Your midwife will arrive with what she needs to assist you to have your baby at home, and monitor you with a hand-held device throughout the proceedings.

Water birth This is increasingly popular, and research suggests that it can benefit you and your baby. You can hire a birthing pool for your home; some hospitals also have pools, but these must be booked in advance. Check that your midwife is able to undertake this type of delivery as special training is now a professional requirement.

Having your baby at home

If you wish to have your baby at home, your community midwife will support your request allowing you to create your own birth environment. You may also choose an independent midwife to care for you throughout pregnancy and birth, but there will be a charge for this.

Be prepared Even if you are planning a home birth you should also pack a bag to take to the hospital just in case (see pp.72–73). Your midwife will bring a home birth pack with her, but you'll also need to put a few things together at home. Here are some items you may wish to have ready:

★ One or two plastic sheets to protect your bed, floor, or sofa.

★ Soft coverings such as old boil-washed towels and cotton sheets (especially if you are planning a water birth).

★ Music or candles – to create the environment that you want.

★ Any pain relief you've organized, such as a TENS machine, homoeopathic remedies, or a hypnosis tape.

★ A hot water bottle or a heated pad.

★ Aromatherapy oils for the bath (check for safety in pregnancy and labour).

★ Light, energy-rich snacks and refreshing drinks to keep you going.

★ Rubbish sacks for dirty linen.

★ Kitchen foil (in case of an emergency where you need to keep your baby warm until the midwife arrives).

★ A container for the placenta.

★ A bucket – in case you need to be sick.

★ A clean, front-opening top for skin-to-skin contact and easier breastfeeding after the birth.

★ Your birth plan; your midwife may end up being someone new, and it's best to have everything written down for her.

★ A warm blanket to keep you cosy after the exertion of giving birth.

★ Your midwife will bring a home birth kit, but in the event that your labour is especially quick and your baby arrives before the midwife, it is advisable to have a few items items. You will need a sterilized pair of sharp kitchen scissors to cut the cord, and something to clamp or tie it off with (such as a new shoe lace).

Pain relief options

Although giving birth is the most natural process in the world, there is no doubt that it can be uncomfortable. Being prepared, and knowing your options will boost your confidence. There is absolutely no shame in getting help with the pain. The most important thing is to bring a healthy baby into the world.

Positive visualization

Take time to learn some positive visualization exercises, which have been proven to help deal with pain and keep you in a healthy frame of mind.

★ Imagine a whoosh of water with every contraction, as your baby moves towards life outside the womb.

★ Imagine the pain as stimulation for your baby, encouraging him to breathe.

★ Visualize your every breath as filling your baby with the oxygen of life.

★ Try to concentrate on visualizing your body opening easily and smoothly, to allow your baby into the world.

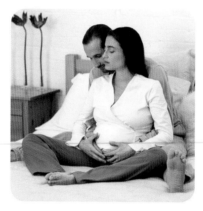

The early stages Slowly inhale through your nose and exhale through your mouth throughout each contraction. Take quicker, shallower breaths as they intensify, then at the peak, breathe only through your mouth.

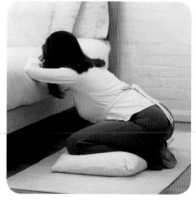

Changing positions Adjusting positions can alter the shape of the pelvis, which helps your baby's head move to the optimal position during the first stage of labour and aids rotation and descent during the second.

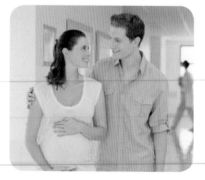

Keeping mobile This speeds up contractions and encourages your baby's head to descend. It also encourages the release of endorphins, which can lift your mood and act as natural pain relief.

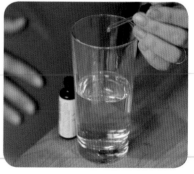

Natural remedies These can be useful during labour, but make sure that you get specialist advice. Remember to consult with your doctor or midwife about anything that you take when you are in labour.

TOP TIP

Learn some natural pain-relieving techniques even if you think you might have an epidural. Deep breathing can really help to get you through the contractions.

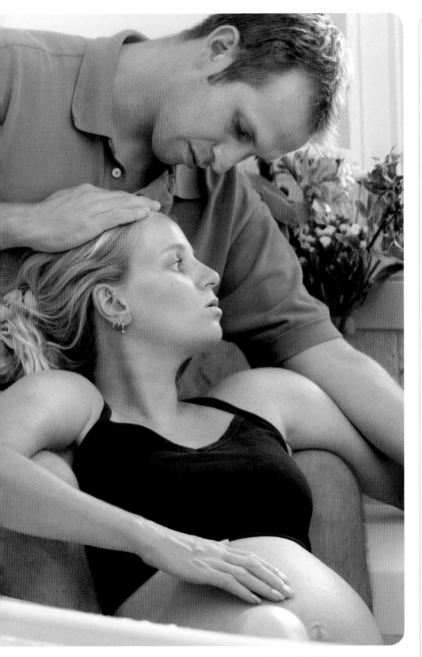

Your main support The contribution that your partner makes to the labour process cannot be underestimated. Whether he jumps into the bath with you, provides massages, and prompts for your breathing exercises, or simply encourages your efforts, he'll need to be involved at every stage. He'll also need to be firmly in tune with your needs, and able to recognize when you need more help, support, or interventions such as pain relief.

Your birth partner's role

Your birth partner will have the honour of being present at this momentous event, but this role does come with some responsibilities.

Involving your partner Talk things through with your partner so that he knows what to do at every stage of labour, and understands how to help. No labour goes exactly according to plan, and it can be a daunting process, but discussing things well in advance will help to keep you positive.

Your birth partner should:
★ Visit your doctor or midwife at least once, to ask his own questions.
★ Join you on your hospital visit.
★ Plan and practise your best route to the hospital.
★ Review your birth plan and identify any areas where compromises can be made.
★ Attend at least one antenatal class, to understand the positions and breathing techniques that will help you through the labour.
★ Have a bag packed with snacks, distractions, massage oils, and anything else that will make the experience more positive for you.
★ Know where your hospital bag is kept, and what may need to be added to it at the last minute.
★ Learn some massage techniques (see p.109).
★ Understand the pain relief on offer, and know how to use any natural remedies and treatments that you want to try.
★ Be prepared. You'll need plenty of love and support, but warn him, however, that there may be times when he may need to back off if you don't want to be touched.

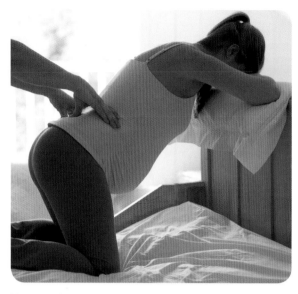

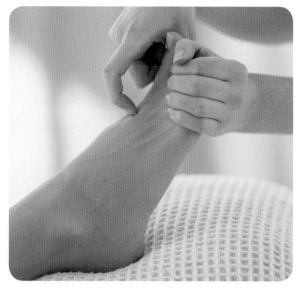

Natural pain relief methods These can include massage (by your partner or a friend), relaxation (which you should learn at antenatal classes), breathing exercises (learned at antenatal classes), water (in a bath, shower, or birthing pool), and gentle exercise. They are all especially effective in the early stages of labour.

Reflexology The manipulation of reflex energy points on your hands and feet is best undertaken by a trained professional, and you'll need to arrange for this. It can help with labour pain, calm you, and encourage contractions by stimulating channels of energy. Your birth partner can use some basic techniques (see p.109).

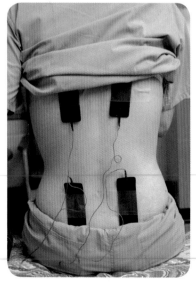

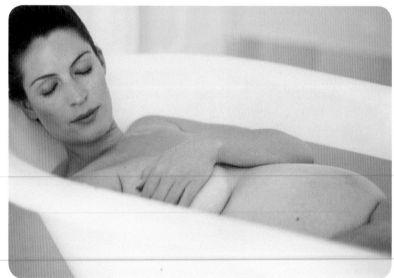

Stimulation TENS (Transcutaneous Electrical Nerve Stimulation) sends a low voltage current that stimulates your body to produce its own pain-relieving substances.

Using water Warm water can be very therapeutic during labour, so make sure you have access to a bath or birthing pool wherever you choose to have your baby. Adding a cup of sea salt to the water will help to prevent your skin from becoming waterlogged and wrinkly, and you can use essential oils (dilute them first in a cup of milk) to enhance the experience.

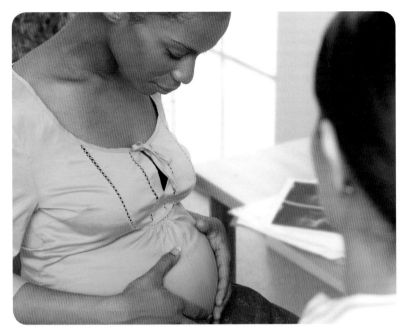

Communicate your feelings Talking to your midwife and your birth partner can help you deal with the discomfort and any fear you may be experiencing. Some women like close physical contact when they are in labour, while others like to be left alone. Don't be afraid to express your needs – and how you are feeling. Your team is there to support you.

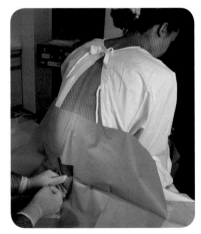

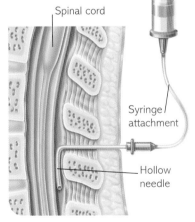

Spinal cord

Syringe attachment

Hollow needle

Epidural anaesthesia This bathes the nerves that run through your lower back, between your uterus and birth canal, with a local anaesthetic. You may have a headache or low blood pressure during and afterwards, but your baby should not be affected.

How an epidural works A fine tube is placed in the region of the nerves (avoiding the spinal cord), and anaesthetic is injected. A standard epidural may make your legs feel "heavy"; but a weaker, "mobile" one will allow some movement.

Other options

There are many other methods, both natural and otherwise, that can be used to help you control the pain of labour, including:

Gas and air Entonox is a pain-relieving mixture of oxygen and nitrous oxide, designed to give pain relief without undue sleepiness. It works in under a minute, and can be used throughout the labour and delivery. Although it crosses the placenta, it has no known effect on babies. Some women feel disorientated, nauseous, dry-mouthed, or light-headed, but it does take the edge off the pain, and you are in complete control of its use.

Pain-killing injections These are a form of pain relief that may only be administered by your midwife or doctor. Pethidine tends to be most often used, as well as Diamorphine and Meptazinol, and these are administered by injecting the muscle of your thigh or bottom. Side-effects can include nausea, vomiting, and drowsiness, and these drugs can also affect your baby's breathing and make him sleepy.

Natural methods There are many types of remedies and therapies available to encourage the process of labour, relieve pain, keep you relaxed, and promote healing. Make sure you get organized in advance, and check that your hospital is happy for you to use them. Acupuncture, for example, is sometimes used in hospitals during labour, and some mothers feel it reduces pain. You will normally visit an acupuncturist in advance of the labour, and then arrange for him or her to treat you during labour.

Your baby's position

There are many different ways that your baby can "present", which is the position in which she is lying in relation to your pelvis. Your baby will alter her position throughout pregnancy, and it is only in the final weeks that this becomes important. Even then it can change in advance of or during labour.

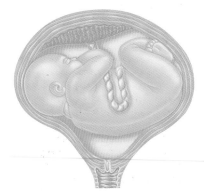

The transverse position This means that the baby is lying across her mother's pelvis. If she does not turn before labour begins, a Caesarean section will be necessary.

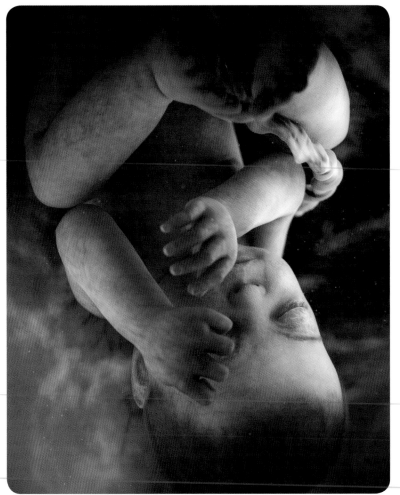

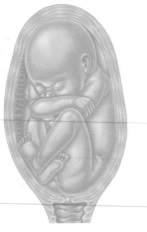

The breech position A breech baby has her bottom rather than her head in the pelvic cavity. A baby can be breech in late pregnancy, but still turn before labour starts.

Head down Here the baby is curled in the fetal position with her head in her mother's pelvis and her chin on her chest: she is in the "vertex" position. Some babies are in this position before labour commences, and others will move into it during labour itself. This is the optimum position for labour, and many babies adopt it just before the big day.

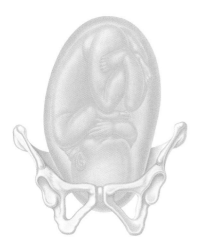

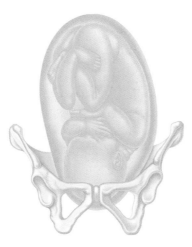

ROP If your baby is facing your front, turned to your right and with her spine along your spine, she is "right posterior". If your baby is in this position in late pregnancy, she may not engage (descend into the pelvis) before labour starts. This means that it is harder for labour to start naturally.

LOP If your baby is slightly to your left, she is "left posterior". With a posterior baby your labour can be longer and you will be aware of pain in your lower back. Babies in this position can be slightly more difficult to deliver and will be born looking up and facing your pubic bone.

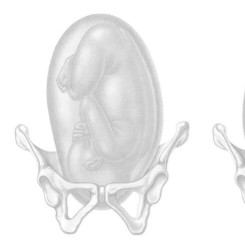

LOA If your baby is facing your back, she is "left anterior". Her spine is curled along the front of your abdomen, or straight up against it. When your baby is in an anterior position, her back feels hard and smooth and rounded on one side of your tummy, and you will normally feel kicks under your ribs. The area around your belly button will feel firm.

ROA If her position is slightly to your right, she is "right anterior". Anterior is ideal because your baby is lined up so as to fit through your pelvis as easily as possible. In this position, your baby's head is easily "flexed", which means that her chin is tucked onto her chest, so that the smallest part of her head will be applied to the cervix first.

Your baby during labour

Childbirth is a natural process, and your baby will not experience pain during labour. She may, however, become tired and distressed if your labour is long or she's in a difficult position.

Presentation As your baby's head presses down on your cervix during labour, the pressure of the contractions encourages her to assume the position in which the smallest possible diameter of her head comes first – or "presents". This doesn't always happen though, and your baby may go through your pelvis facing up or turned sideways.

Head "moulding" Her head will change shape during labour. The bones of her skull are not yet fused, and are free to move, allowing her head to "mould" to the size and shape of your pelvic opening.

Ready to breathe Your baby will continue to receive her oxygen from your placenta, via her umbilical cord, but during labour your baby's lungs begin to dry out so that they expand to take in air when she is delivered and the umbilical cord is cut (once it has stopped pulsating).

Temperature control Your baby's thyroid gland helps her to adjust from the hotter temperature of your womb to the cooler delivery room.

Monitoring Your baby's progress will be monitored by your midwife or doctor (see pp.110–11) to ensure swift intervention if she should become too distressed or exhausted.

When a baby is overdue

It's not uncommon for babies to take their time to arrive, and your doctor or midwife may decide that it is best to get things going. Induction is intended simply to kickstart your labour, after which it should be as normal as possible.

Late babies

Try not to panic. Although it can seem rather unnatural to use medication to start your labour, if things go on for too long, it really is the best option.

Be patient It is very unusual for babies to appear on their due dates, and with first-time mums it can be another two weeks before anything gets going. If your pregnancy is progressing well, and your baby is continuing to thrive, your midwife will probably be happy to leave things, and let nature take its course. If nothing has happened by about week 41, you may need to be induced.

The safe option The reason for this is that there is a concern that "post maturity" (going past your dates) can pose a risk to your baby. A very small number of babies die unexpectedly while still in the uterus at 42 weeks, and this number increases again at 43 weeks. It is very rare for this to happen, but induction is a precaution that most medical professionals and mothers-to-be wish to take. Over time, your placenta becomes less efficient, and you may not be able to keep up with the demands placed on your body. Some women's bodies simply never get the message to get things going, and induction is the only way.

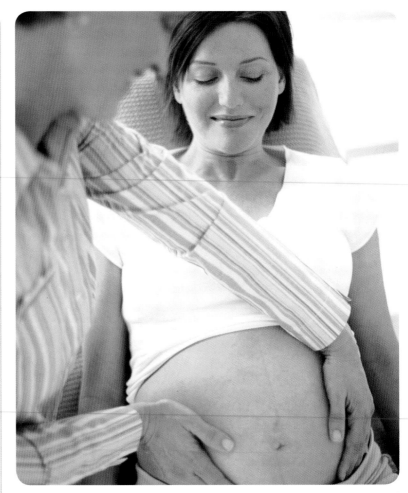

40 weeks Once you pass this mark, you will see your doctor or midwife weekly until your baby arrives. If there are no signs of labour, induction may be necessary. A membrane sweep is often the first step, and it involves the midwife inserting a finger into your cervix, stretching it, and then making a firm, circular, sweeping motion around the inside to separate your cervix from the membranes of the sac holding your baby. Labour will often start naturally within 48 hours, but be prepared, the procedure can be uncomfortable.

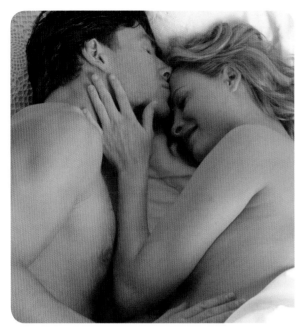

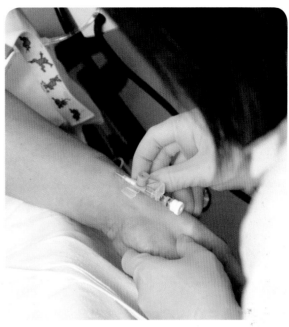

A natural start Sexual intercourse can help to get things going, so if you are concerned about induction, you can give this a try. Orgasm may stimulate the uterus into action, and sex can encourage the release of oxytocin, which stimulates contractions. Semen also contains prostaglandins, which can soften your cervix in preparation for dilation. Sex is safe as long as your waters have not broken.

Induction If a membrane sweep has failed, synthetic hormonal induction may be required (see below) to bring about contractions. Your doctor or midwife may undertake an "amniotomy" (break your waters manually) either with an "amniohook" (a crochet-type hook) or an "amnicot" (a glove with a pricked end on one finger), which they will place in your vagina to rupture the amniotic membrane.

Synthetic hormonal stimulants

In some cases, your midwife may decide that your waters should be broken manually to get things started. If this doesn't work, however, and a membrane sweep – and anything else you may have tried – are ineffective, you'll probably need some drug intervention:

Prostaglandin This hormone is used to ripen the cervix. There are two forms: you are given a tablet to take orally, or a gel or pessary (a small, bullet-shaped oil-based lozenge, containing a hormonal stimulant) is placed in the vagina. You are normally asked to call the maternity unit early in the morning and may be given a pessary first thing, then if nothing has happened, another, six hours later. Prostaglandin gels and pessaries can be uncomfortable, and you can experience strong cramping.

Oxytocin Offered to stimulate contractions, this is used either in conjunction with prostaglandins, or afterwards. Given by continuous intravenous injection, your baby and uterus will be monitored during the process, and the dose increased until your labour is progressing well.

Stalled or slow labour Oxytocin is also used to encourage labour that has ground to a halt, or is progressing too slowly as it can encourage stronger, more frequent contractions. However, these can seem very painful without the gradual build-up that most women experience. If you find it very uncomfortable, practise your breathing and consider some of the pain-relief options on offer. You may find that a little gas and air will take the edge off the pain. A warm bath can also help.

Monitoring You and your baby will be electronically monitored (see pp.110–11) throughout induction to check that it is effective and that you are both coping well.

What happens during labour

Although the process is the same for all mothers – and babies – labour can progress at different rates, so help may be needed to keep you going.

Arriving at the hospital

Most women like to wait as long as possible before heading to the hospital, experiencing the first hours of stage-one labour in the comfort of their own home.

Phone first Call your maternity unit on the direct line listed in your maternity notes (which you should take with you). Phone in advance of your arrival so that they can check whether you are in labour and make the necessary preparations.

Initial assessment When you arrive, a midwife will establish your EDD, whether you have had a "show" (see p.103), and if your waters have broken, as well as the nature, length, and intensity of your contractions.

Thorough check Your midwife will check your temperature, pulse and respiration, blood pressure, and urine, and feel and palpate your abdomen to check your baby's position. She'll perform a vaginal examination to see how far your cervix has dilated and listen to your baby's heart rate after a contraction.

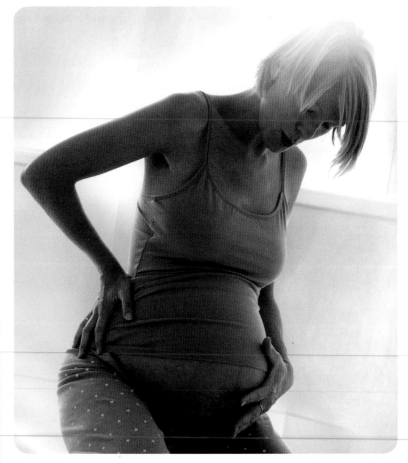

Pre-labour "Effacement" of the cervix is when the neck of the cervix, which leads from the uterus to your vagina, starts to soften and shorten. Signs of pre-labour can include the loss of your mucus plug (see p.103), grumbling pains in your back or abdomen, and feeling queasy. This stage can take as long as a few days, so don't head for the hospital just yet.

The dilation of your cervix and the process of labour

Throughout pregnancy, your cervix is closed and sealed with a plug of mucus, to prevent infection. In the first stage of labour, your cervix has to open, to allow your baby to be born. In the days or even weeks before the birth, your cervix will begin to soften and shorten.

The beginning We do not know exactly what starts labour, but it may be triggered by hormones produced by your baby's adrenal gland that encourage your uterus to contract. If you are induced, hormones are administered to stimulate contractions (see p.99). Contractions open your cervix and help to push your baby down the birth canal (vagina). As your cervix dilates (opens) contractions come closer together and last longer, so labour gets progressively faster. It usually takes longer to get from being 1 or 2cm dilated to 5 or 6cm, than it does to get from 5cm to full dilation (approximately 10cm).

The descent As your cervix slowly opens, you will experience some pain.

It helps to stay mobile at this stage, to encourage your baby's descent.

Your baby's position This will affect how efficiently your cervix dilates. If your baby is in the posterior position, the front of his head rather than his crown will press against your cervix, which slows down the process a little.

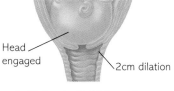

Head engaged / 2cm dilation

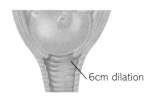

6cm dilation

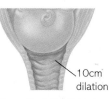

10cm dilation

1 **At the start of labour,** the cervix thins and gradually dilates (opens). This may take some time and your contractions will be irregular.

2 **Over the next eight to 18 hours** (on average), your cervix dilates completely to allow your baby's head and body to descend.

3 **At the end of the first stage,** your cervix will be fully dilated, contractions are continuous, and you will nearly be ready to push.

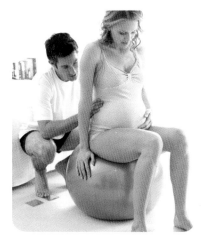

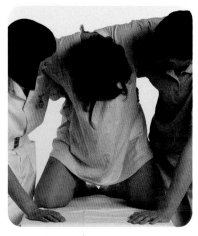

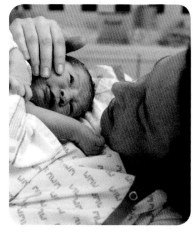

First stage The longest stage, it is usually between 14 and 18 hours for a first delivery, and eight to 14 hours for subsequent births. Contractions become stronger and closer together as your baby descends.

Second stage This involves you pushing your baby down through your birth canal and into the world. Your midwife will guide you, to help you work with your natural instincts and reduce the risk of tearing.

Third stage You will have your new baby in your arms, but must now deliver the placenta. With your consent you may have an injection of oxytocin to speed up this phase and lessen the risk of heavy bleeding.

Am I in labour?

As your pregnancy progresses, you may experience Braxton Hicks' "practice" contractions. These can easily be mistaken for the real thing, so before you go to hospital make sure that all the signs are there.

When to get help

While labour can last at least a few hours (and often much, much longer) for most first-time mums, some women do experience fast births.

Don't panic No matter how you are feeling, making the effort to stay calm will help your labour progress. Phone your maternity unit:

★ If your contractions come thick and fast, or you experience a strong urge to push – you need to get to hospital immediately.

★ Your waters break, either as a sudden gush, or a slow trickle.

★ Your baby moves less than usual.

★ You have any vaginal bleeding that is not associated with your mucus plug being discharged (blood-tinged mucus).

★ You have a fever, changes in your vision, severe headaches, or abdominal (or diaphragm) pain.

★ You experience sharp, stabbing, or unusual pains of any description, or feel faint or dizzy.

★ While childbirth can be very uncomfortable, there is usually a gradual build up of pain. Any sudden pain should be investigated.

★ If you can feel any sensation that may lead you to believe that your baby's head is emerging, call an ambulance immediately.

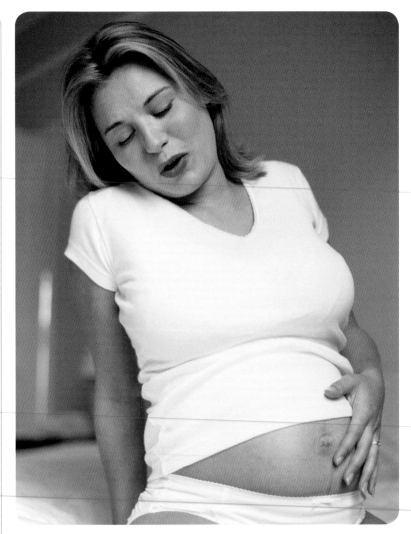

The "latent" phase Although this is early labour, it is still part of the first stage, so you may experience some cramping, much like strong menstrual cramps, and some pain in your back or abdomen. Don't be surprised if they stop for a while though; this is normal.

Signs that you may be in labour

In conjunction with other symptoms, a strong nesting urge may be a sign that things have commenced. Try to resist giving into it, even if it does seem inexplicably urgent to iron the pillowcases. You'll need to save your energy for the hours and days to come.

Be prepared Thinking that labour has begun and going to the maternity unit only to be sent home can be disappointing, but the number of false alarms you have doesn't matter, the important thing is that you and your baby are safe. Most women experience some of the symptoms listed here, but you may not experience all of them. Try to remember that early labour does not always progress at a steady pace, so you may experience a run of strong contractions followed by a period of relative inactivity. Make use of these intervals to get some rest.

Common signs of labour include:
★ A profuse emptying of the bowels, vomiting, or nausea just before your body swings into action.

★ Lower back pain.
★ Regular contractions that become increasingly close together and painful (although don't be surprised if they stop; this is normal, too).
★ A "show" (losing your mucus plug – the collection of mucus that plugs the cervix; this can be blood-stained).
★ Your waters breaking, which can occur as a slow drip, or a rush (don't be alarmed by the quantity of water – there's a lot in there).
★ If contractions come and go over a long period, you probably aren't there yet; when you are in labour there should be a distinct pattern. If, however, the stopping and starting is accompanied by other symptoms, it's a good idea to call your midwife for advice.

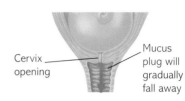

Cervix opening — Mucus plug will gradually fall away

1 As your labour approaches, your cervix softens in response to the prostaglandin hormones that are released into your bloodstream.

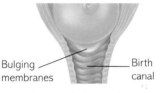

Bulging membranes — Birth canal

2 The amniotic membrane is bulging through the cervix and may be about to break (waters breaking) so labour may be imminent or have already started. The amniotic fluid may come out as a gush or just a trickle.

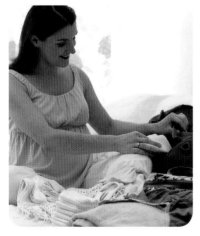

Get ready When you experience regular contractions, put any last-minute items such as drinks and snacks in your hospital bag. Then relax. Most labours – particularly for first-time mums – take a while to get going.

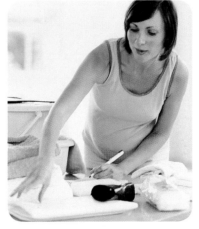

Staying at home If you are planning to give birth at home, and you think that labour has begun, get everything ready for your midwife's arrival (see p.91). Remain calm, have a rest, and something to eat.

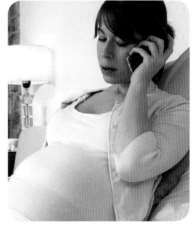

Important calls Phone your partner, the maternity unit or birthing centre, and/or your midwife when you experience regular contractions – your care-givers will need some advance warning.

The first stage of labour

There are two distinct phases of the first stage of labour: early labour and active labour, and it may take some time to progress through them.

What happens

★ First, your cervix has to soften and shorten. This can occur in the days or even weeks before you go into labour.

★ Contractions will begin to gradually push your baby from your uterus down through the birth canal.

★ These contractions generally come closer together, each one lasts longer, and they feel more intense.

★ Your cervix dilates from a closed position to about 10cm when it is considered to be fully dilated.

★ Although you may have had a show, contractions and possibly broken waters, you are not considered to be in established labour until your cervix has dilated to at least 3cm.

★ It can take up to 14 hours (or more) for your cervix to become fully dilated.

★ It is usual to have one contraction every 10 minutes or so at the outset of labour, increasing to contractions every 30 seconds or so at the end. Early in the process, contractions will last about 40 or 50 seconds; by the end of the first stage they will last more than a minute. All of this acts to push your baby out of your uterus and into the world.

★ The end of the first stage is called "transition". It can be the most difficult period of labour, lasting for an hour or so, with very intense contractions.

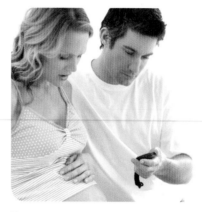

Time contractions When contractions begin, start timing them. When they form a pattern, and become more frequent, you can be sure that you are in early labour.

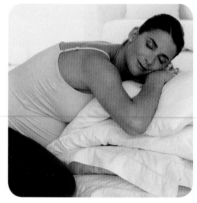

Rest Although you may feel excited by the impending birth, try to rest, and find an upright position in the early stages of labour to keep things moving in a positive direction.

The station

You may hear your midwife mention your "station".

Engaged The "station" is the degree to which your baby's head is engaged as she moves into your pelvis. When the top of her head (or another part of her body, if she is in another position) arrives at the level of your ischial spines (bony prominences about halfway down your pelvis), she is said to be at "0" station or "engaged". She may engage before going into labour, and may be at station "-1", "0", or even "+1" when it begins.

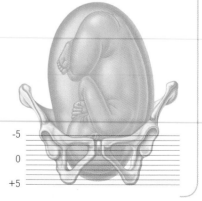

-5
0
+5

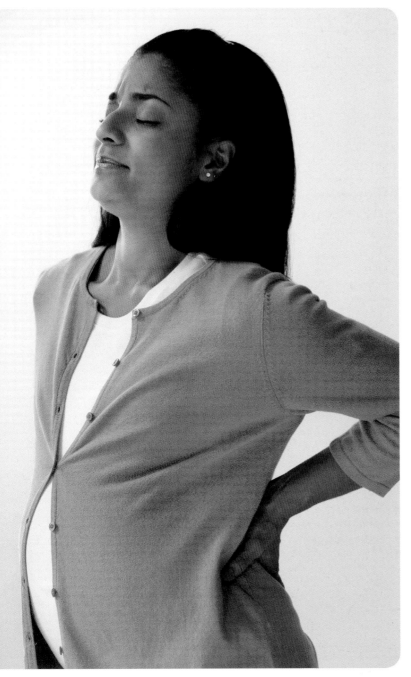

Keep moving Even the earliest contractions can be surprisingly uncomfortable, but a slow progression towards more frequent, intense contractions gives you a chance to adjust. Try to keep mobile; it will keep things going, and gravity will encourage your baby's descent.

Your emotional state

You may find that your emotions swing dramatically during labour. You may feel elated at the outset, but it's also normal to experience anxiety, as the reality suddenly hits home.

Keep calm Each stage of labour comes with its own physical and emotional challenges, and it's important that you keep things in perspective. In the early stages, it is important to relax in a safe and comfortable environment. Get plenty of support from your birth partner, and keep yourself occupied until you really need to concentrate.

Stay focused When active labour begins, many women can feel shocked and out of control. Remember that your breathing will help you to work through the contractions, and that you do have options for pain relief. When you feel like giving up, imagine your new baby in your arms and aim for that positive outcome. Practising relaxation techniques and positive visualization can do wonders for calming your emotions.

Don't worry Some women feel angry and irritated during labour. This is normal, and the result of stress, the hormones circulating around your body, and your heightened emotional state. Many women are uncharacteristically rude – even swearing or shouting at their birth partners. Try to remember that you are under intense physical and emotional pressure, and all will be forgotten in a few hours' time.

Positions for early labour

Staying mobile and adopting a position that is comfortable for you can go a long way towards getting things going – and relieving discomfort.

Working through the experience

Childbirth can be a long, slow process, so involve both your birth partner and your midwife as much as you can. As things progress, remember to:

Relax Go with the rhythm of your contractions, and try to imagine what your baby is doing as he rotates into your pelvis, and his head pushes down on your cervix.

Breathe Continue breathing slowly and fully between contractions, and in a relaxed and regular manner as they occur. To slow things down and make sure that you get a deep lungful of air, breathe in through your nose for five seconds and out through your mouth for seven. You may wish to alter your breathing as your labour progresses (see p.92).

Trust yourself Your body has been in training for this event for nine months; the hormone relaxin has softened the ligaments in your pelvis to make them more flexible and your baby's head will also adjust in size to fit through the gap.

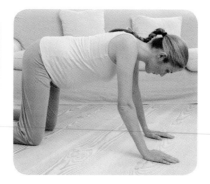

On all fours Kneel like this if you feel tired or experience backache. This is good if your baby is posterior, as it shifts his weight away from your spine. It's also ideal during delivery, to reduce the risk of tearing, and if you need a break from intense contractions.

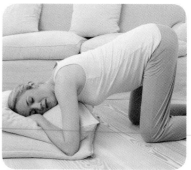

Soft support Kneeling and leaning forwards onto cushions with your bottom raised helps to ease backache – particularly useful if your baby is in the posterior position. It can also help during transition, when you need to resist the urge to push.

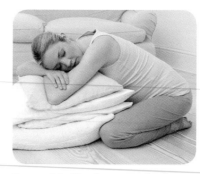

Rest upright Kneeling over a pile of pillows or cushions on the floor can create an upright position to encourage your baby's descent. You could also move your hips back and forth, to loosen things up.

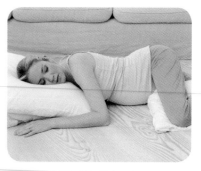

Recharge Lie on your side with your knees bent and pillows supporting your leg between contractions. Staying active will speed things up, but you will also need to recharge your batteries from time to time.

Sitting upright Leaning against a chair (facing forward and astride) can help to relax your pelvic floor muscles. This position will also make use of gravity and increase your pelvic opening by approximately 28 per cent.

Staying positive

Although labour can sometimes seem like a marathon, staying positive and working through the stages of labour with confidence will not only make the experience more rewarding, but also more comfortable.

Positive pain

We are conditioned to think of pain as a message that there is something wrong, but labour pain is positive pain with a positive outcome. So relax into the experience:

Don't panic Try not to become tense or frightened, as both of these responses trigger the release of adrenalin in your body, which can increase the intensity of pain. Panicking can affect your breathing, which robs your body of the oxygen it needs to perform effectively.

It is bearable One study found that only about 20 per cent of women found labour "horrible" or "excruciating", and another 20 per cent said that they had low levels of pain, with the rest somewhere in the middle. While the discomfort is very real, it helps to remember that women have been having babies since the dawn of time. It's also worth noting that the women who rate their birth experiences the most highly are not necessarily those who had the least painful birth.

Work through it Use all of the techniques you've learned to work through the pain, and see every contraction as one more step towards holding your much-loved baby in your arms at last.

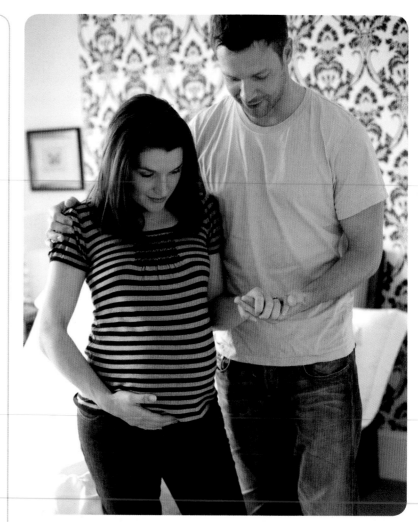

Ask for support Sharing the experience and being encouraged through the process will make things much easier. It's also important to remain as mobile as possible, particularly in the first stage of labour. Keeping active is one productive step you can take towards getting your baby in your arms; it will also help to lift your spirits.

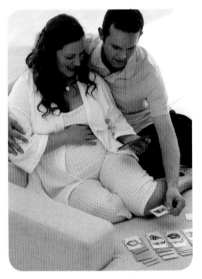

Stay together Spend time with your partner; distracting yourself from the process with a long walk, a DVD, or a board game will help get you through the early stages. Better still, take a nap together. You may have a long night ahead of you.

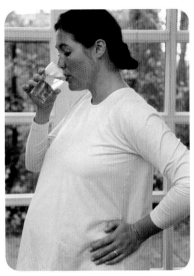

Keep hydrated Drink plenty of fresh water to keep you hydrated throughout labour; there is some evidence that cramping is worse when dehydration sets in. It's also important to eat a light, nutritious meal that will see you through the process.

Tips to get things going

Many labours grind to a halt just when you think you are well on your way. Try not to be disillusioned or frustrated; instead, focus on positively visualizing the birth of your baby, and try these tips:

A brisk walk You may not feel particularly energetic, but walking across rough terrain can do a lot to help shift your baby downwards, and so stimulate contractions.

Try reflexology Ask your partner to firmly squeeze your second and third toes (the first toe being your big toe), releasing, and then repeating, simultaneously. This is thought to directly affect your uterus.

Massage Some simple techniques can help to ease discomfort. Relaxation can encourage the labour process, and massage is a wonderful way to achieve this. Choose an aromatherapy oil such as lavender, which is an adaptogen; this means that it will work on a number of levels, stimulating you or relaxing you when you need it.

Think positive If you feel anxious, simply say to yourself: "I can do this. My healthy baby is on her way. I am strong and able to work through these contractions".

Ask a friend Chat with a friend who had a really good birth experience; not only will you find it reassuring, but it will fill you with the self-belief that you can do it, too. Confidence and a positive frame of mind are associated with successful, less painful labours.

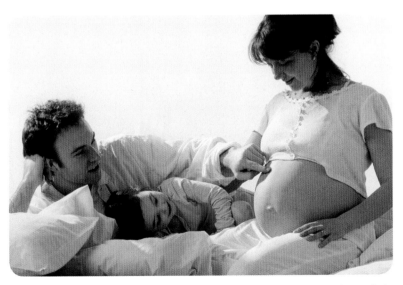

Relax with your family Being at home for as long as you can manage may make you feel more secure and less anxious. If pains become intense, it may be a good idea to have your other children looked after by someone else, so that they do not become frightened by the experience; however, while you are still comfortable enough to chat you can involve them in the process. They'll be excited to know that their new sibling is finally on the way.

Monitoring

When labour has been properly established, you and your baby will be regularly monitored by your midwife or doctor to check that all is progressing as it should, and that you are both managing the process successfully.

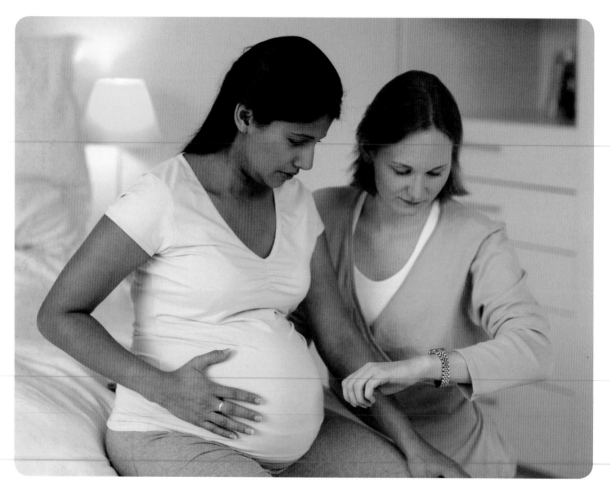

Timing your contractions This is the first step in monitoring the progress of your labour. As your cervix gradually opens and your baby heads down the birth canal, they will become closer together and more intense. Contractions can, however, stop and start from time to time – even when labour has been established. If this is what happens in your case, you may require a little intervention in the form of an oxytocin drip to get things moving again (see p.99). A prolonged labour is not ideal for you or your baby.

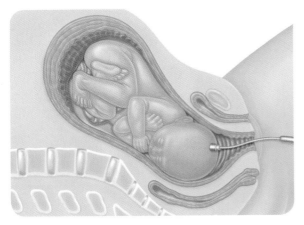

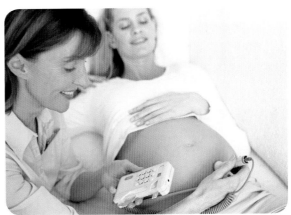

Electronic fetal monitoring (EFM) If your pregnancy is classified as "high risk" a small electrode can be clipped to your baby's scalp (or her bottom, if she is breech), to pick up and transmit her heartbeat (see below) and check for signs of distress. The digital read-out will change constantly, so don't panic.

"Mobile" monitoring If you are "low risk" and wish to avoid being strapped to an external fetal monitoring machine, your midwife can listen to your baby's heartbeat using a hand-held device. She'll usually do this every 15 minutes or so after each contraction, and every five minutes during the second stage.

How external fetal monitoring is done

During labour your baby's heartbeat and your contractions will be measured by electronic sensors placed on the top of your abdomen and over your baby's heart. Wires connect to a machine that produces a print-out of the readings, known as a "cardiotocograph".

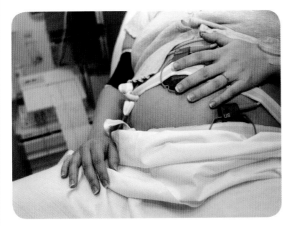

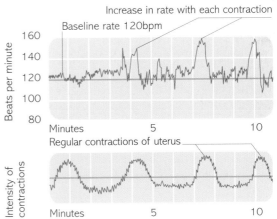

Heartbeat Your baby's heartbeat will be recorded against a "baseline" measurement of 110–120 beats per minute (see right, top). Her heart rate will rise and fall when you have contractions, and this is absolutely normal. Your midwife will be looking for a variation in the pattern, which could indicate distress.

Contractions These will be recorded to see how long they last and how often they occur. If your cervix is not dilating, you may need help to strengthen your contractions (see p.99). The monitor will be used throughout labour if your pregnancy is high risk, or you have an epidural, but only intermittently if all is well.

Labour aids

There is a variety of tools and techniques that you can use to increase your comfort during labour. Many women find it useful to keep busy, to distract them from any discomfort, and using aids goes a long way to achieving that.

Homeopathic remedies for labour

Homeopathy is not only safe during pregnancy and while breastfeeding, but research has found that it can be very effective in encouraging a shorter, more positive birth experience. See a registered homeopath who can put together a kit for you, or consider some of the following remedies:

★ Aconite for dealing with panic, restlessness, and fear.

★ Arnica to keep you going through a tiring labour and help relieve pain. You could take Arnica 30c every hour once labour is established, and after the birth for afterpains and to encourage healing.

★ Calendula to encourage healing after a tear, episiotomy, or Caesarean section.

★ Caulophyllum when labour doesn't progress or stops, or labour pains are ineffective and your cervix is not dilating.

★ Chamomilla for anger, impatience, and unbearable pain that makes you feel as if you want to give up.

★ Gelsemium for anxiety, with shivering and visual disturbances.

★ Kali carb for backache in labour, or if your baby is in a "posterior" position (see p.97).

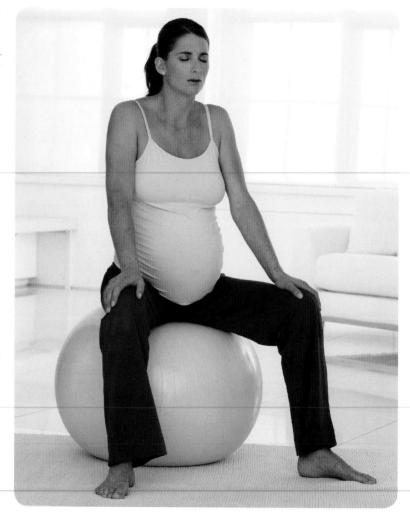

A birthing ball Ideal for relieving discomfort during pregnancy and birth, a ball provides a firm, yet comfortable place to sit, and encourages good posture. During labour, you can sit on the ball (you could lean against a wall for support) and gently rock and sway your hips to move your baby down the birth canal by subtly adjusting the position of your pelvis.

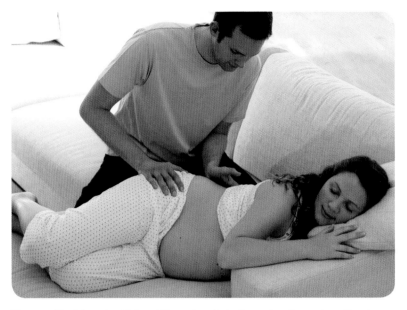

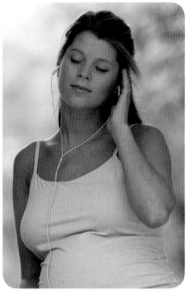

Massage Used throughout labour, this can be a fantastic way to relieve pain and tension, and encourage a more positive frame of mind. You may wish to use some aromatherapy oils to enhance the process. Some of the best are lavender (pain relieving, muscle relaxant, and antidepressant) and Roman chamomile (anti-inflammatory and emotionally soothing).

Music Favourite songs can be of enormous benefit during labour. You could choose something soothing at first perhaps, and a few dance tracks when things get tough.

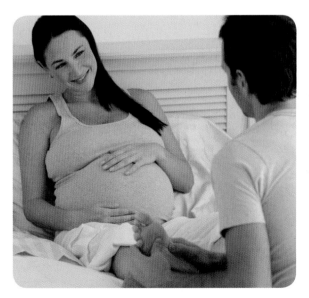

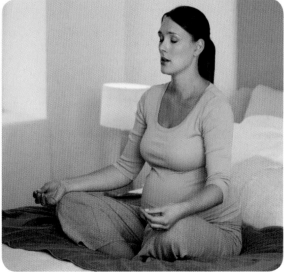

Foot massage Some simple techniques can be used in early labour to encourage relaxation and offer pain relief. You need to know how, though, so it's a good idea to encourage your birth partner to get a few tips from a registered reflexologist in advance.

HypnoBirthing This involves being taught simple self-hypnosis, relaxation, and breathing techniques. You'll be awake and alert throughout your labour (not in a trance), and advocates claim that the deep relaxation reduces pain, tension, fear, and anxiety.

The second stage of labour

The second stage of labour will begin when your cervix is fully dilated, and is the point where you can take charge and push your baby into the world.

Water birth

If you are in the care of a midwife who is experienced in dealing with water births, it is perfectly possible to deliver your baby in the water.

Staying safe Whether you use a birthing pool, or even a large bath, your baby will not drown, as he will still be connected to the umbilical cord and receiving an oxygenated supply of blood via the placenta.

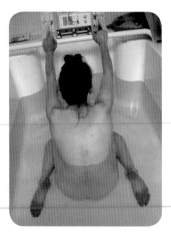

Beneficial There is evidence that many women have a less painful and more comfortable labour in water.

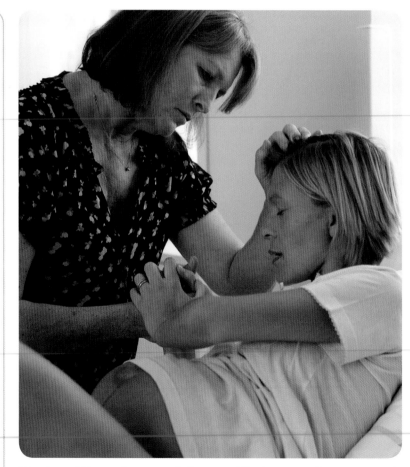

Take charge This second stage can take from around 30 minutes to two hours or more, and can be physically exhausting, particularly after a long first stage. You midwife will encourage you to go with your natural instincts and bear down when you feel the urge. Your birth partner's support is absolutely crucial at this time as you take charge of delivering your baby.

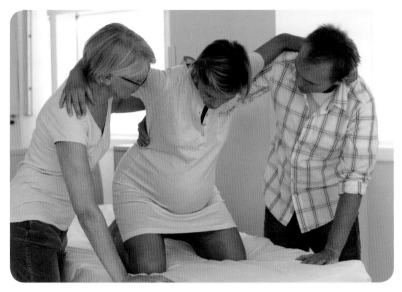

Get comfortable With the help of your midwife and your birth partner, find a position that feels right for you. Staying upright allows you to use the force of gravity to help get your baby out. You may become tired, so lean on your helpers.

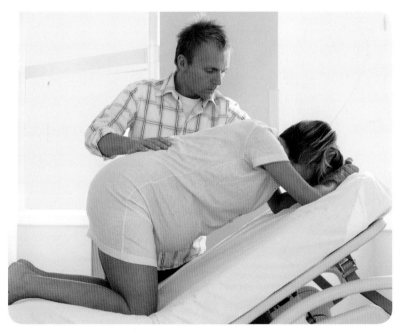

Stay upright Research shows that women who give birth upright or in the all-fours position have less pain in labour and birth, have shorter labours and pushing times, less shoulder dystocia (where the baby's shoulders get stuck in the pelvis), and fewer perineal tears.

What your birth partner can do

The role of your birth partner cannot be underestimated, particularly in the second stage of labour when you have to work hard to physically expel your baby down the birth canal.

Your partner will need to:

★ Know what is in your birth plan, to be sure that you and your baby are treated as you wish.

★ Be emotionally supportive and encouraging – your partner should ideally maintain eye contact.

★ Keep you relaxed between contractions with massage, labour aids, and distractions.

★ Offer any natural remedies that will help you to get through each stage, and keep a careful check on your pain management.

★ Help you to find a comfortable position, and make suggestions when things aren't working.

★ Encourage you to take deep breaths as you push.

★ Distract you when you need to stop pushing or resist bearing down.

★ Ask for help when you need it, or speak up for you if you are finding things difficult to cope with.

★ Make sure you get enough to drink and eat; you may not feel like eating anything, but you will need to stay hydrated to keep going. Small sips of water or ice cubes can help.

★ Offer you some glucose tablets or an isotonic sports drink if you are running out of energy.

★ Possibly hold a mirror to your vagina when your baby crowns. It will be your first sight of your baby.

★ Perhaps cut the cord.

★ Most importantly, offer love, support, and encouragement.

The final push

The second stage of labour involves pushing your baby out into the world. You may experience several strong urges to push. With each push, your baby will move a little further down the birth canal on her way to meet you.

Tips for the second stage of labour

★ Empty your bladder, as this can make pushing out your baby much easier.

★ Try to stay upright – the force of gravity can make pushing more efficient.

★ Try not to hold your breath when you are pushing – your body needs plenty of oxygen to do the job efficiently.

★ If you are tired or have an epidural in place, lie on your left-hand side – this improves your circulation, takes the pressure off your back, and helps to open up your pelvis.

★ Listen to your midwife's instructions; she'll help you to time your pushes to make sure they coincide with contractions.

★ Change position often – this can help to shift your baby's position, and move her along the birth canal.

★ Practise your breathing between contractions to stay calm and focused.

TOP TIP
Listen to your midwife, who will be monitoring the position of your baby. She may ask you to pant, rather than push, to encourage your body to open up gradually.

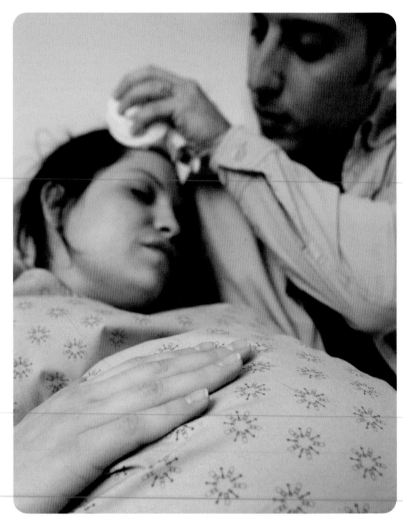

Coping with contractions You can expect contractions to occur roughly two or three minutes apart (or even more frequently), and they will last about a minute. This can seem like a long time when you are exhausted, but work with your natural instincts and use every ounce of energy you have to bear down as each contraction occurs.

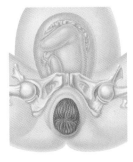

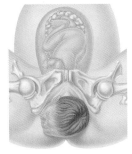

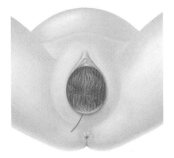

Crowning When your baby's head is fully visible it is known as "crowning" and marks the beginning of the second stage. As the head presses down on your pelvic floor it creates an urge to push or "bear down".

Head delivery As your womb continues to contract and you begin to push, your baby's head will be delivered, little by little. If the cord is around your baby's neck or body your midwife will unravel it as she is born.

Birth of your baby Next your baby's body will be delivered, usually fairly quickly. Your midwife may turn your baby slightly to help her shoulders negotiate with the next contraction.

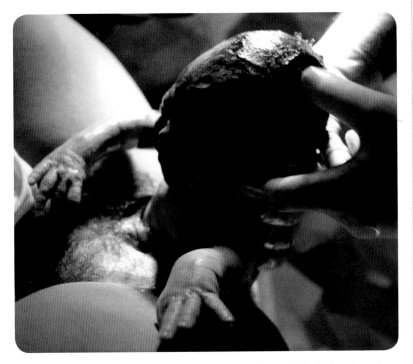

Giving birth Finding a comfortable, upright position can help to make the birth easier as the pull of gravity will make your contractions more effective. Moving around can also speed up the proceedings. But don't exhaust yourself – this stage can last for up to three hours. You may feel that you want to lie down to deliver your baby and your midwife will be happy to assist you in this position. The most important thing is to relax, and listen to your body.

Episiotomy and perineal tears

About two-thirds of women will need stitches as a result of giving birth.

When to cut Once your baby has crowned, it may be necessary to widen the vaginal opening and make delivery easier. If your midwife feels that this is necessary (for instance if your baby is in distress and needs to be delivered quickly, or if she thinks that you are in danger of severe tearing) you will be asked for your consent to an episiotomy – a small cut in the perineum. Episiotomies and large tears will need to be stitched, but small tears may be left to heal naturally. A local anaesthetic is administered before stitching, so you should not experience any pain.

Recovery After the birth, you may have some discomfort as the site heals. Pouring warm water over your perineum as you urinate can help to ease discomfort, and painkillers and cooling pads can also reduce pain. Most wounds feel better after a few weeks, although episiotomies can take a little longer to heal.

Episiotomy This involves making a cut in the muscular area between your vagina and back passage.

First moments of life

The moment your baby is placed on your chest your life changes, and even the most difficult labour will fade from your memory as you greet your new arrival.

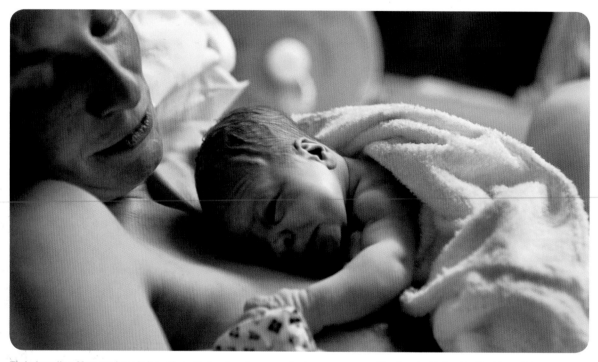

Early bonding Your newborn baby will usually be placed on your chest as soon as possible after the birth – ideally skin to skin – to encourage the bonding process and to help establish breastfeeding. He may begin to root around quite quickly in search of your breast and begin suckling. Enjoy this moment of calm and take the time to reflect on your extraordinary achievement.

How your newborn may look

You may be a little shocked at first that your newborn baby looks nothing like you imagined. Don't be surprised if his head is elongated or moulded or if his eyes and genitals are puffy and his nose squashed. Within 24 hours the visible signs of the trauma of birth will have disappeared.

Skin Your newborn may be covered in a white, waxy substance, known as vernix, which has protected his skin in the uterus. He may also have blood, amniotic fluid, and patches of green meconium on his skin and nails. Premature babies may be covered with fine hair, known as lanugo. Many babies are born with birthmarks, such as stork bites (on the eyelids and the nape of the neck), which fade over time.

Hair Some babies are born with hair, some not; the colour isn't relevant at this stage.

Eyes Your baby's eye colour may change in the months after the birth.

After a water birth If you have delivered your baby in water, you may wish to stay in the birthing pool until your baby's cord has been clamped and cut, and then deliver your placenta on "dry land".

Assisted births

Some births simply don't go to plan, and if you are exhausted or your baby is becoming distressed, you may need a little help to get her out into the world. The two main methods of assisting delivery are using forceps and a ventouse, and each has its advantages and disadvantages.

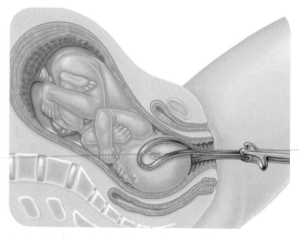

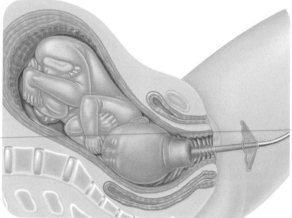

Forceps These are large stainless-steel tongs with ends that curve around your baby's head to help extract her from your womb. They have a good success rate, and pose little risk, although your baby may experience some bruising, and you will probably need an episiotomy (see p.117), which may leave you uncomfortable after the birth.

Ventouse This delivery involves positioning a silicone plastic cap on your baby's head, and extracting the air with a vacuum. When you have a contraction, you'll be asked to push, while your doctor or midwife pulls. This is not as traumatic as forceps, but you may still require an episiotomy. It can also cause swelling to your baby's head.

Why do I need an assisted birth?

Although many women put a "no forceps" note on their birth plans, it is worth considering the fact that some assistance may be necessary. In advance of the birth you may wish to ask your midwife if you can choose which method is used should it be required. You may need assistance if:

★ You are absolutely exhausted (perhaps after a very long labour) and unable to continue pushing.
★ Your contractions are too weak to help your baby out.
★ Your baby is in an awkward position.
★ Your baby is suffering some distress and her heartbeat is becoming irregular.
★ Your baby is being born prematurely.

★ Your baby is in the breech position or another position that makes it difficult for her to make an exit (such as face up).
★ Your pelvis is small or shaped in such a way that a normal delivery is difficult.
★ You've had an epidural, which means that you may find it difficult to know how and when to push.
★ You have a very large baby.

Delivery position You may be asked to lie on the bed with your feet in stirrups as this will help the medical team to extract your baby as quickly as possible. An episiotomy (see p.117) may be needed to make room to insert the forceps or ventouse. In most cases you will be offered some sort of pain relief, such as an epidural or spinal block, or a local anaesthetic.

Once your baby is born

A few minutes after your baby is born, her umbilical cord will be clamped and then cut, and if all is well, you'll be given your baby to hold. You may be amazed by the rush of emotions that you experience in those first few moments of motherhood – don't worry if it all seems a little overwhelming.

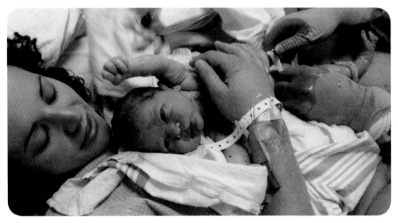

Clamping the cord After the birth, the cord may be left to pulsate for a few minutes, which provides your baby with more blood and oxygen. Clamping may take place with your baby on your chest, as this can stimulate her vital signs (see p.133) and delivery of the placenta.

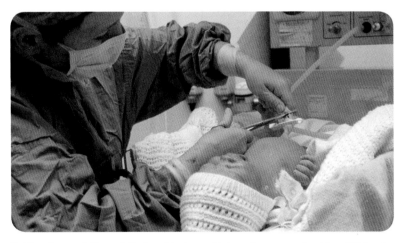

Cutting the cord The umbilical cord is clamped in two places – usually at 1cm (½in) and 4cm (1½in) from your baby's tummy. It will be cut with scissors by your partner or the midwife. At this stage, your placenta is still inside you, and will be delivered in the third stage of labour.

How you may be feeling

New mums find themselves feeling lots of emotions – love, pride, astonishment, achievement, shock, relief – sometimes all at the same time!

Tired and emotional Depending on the length of your labour and any medication you may have been given, you may feel more exhausted than anything else. It's normal to feel a little shaky and tearful, and to experience swings of mood from high to low in the first hours and days after you give birth.

Feeling "empty" For nine long months you've had a little person inside you, sharing your body and defining the way you live your life. Some women find themselves mourning their "bump" and the closeness they achieved with their babies during pregnancy.

Opposite sex If your baby is not the sex you had anticipated, give yourself some time to come to terms with any possible disappointment and focus instead on the fact that your baby is healthy and well. Feelings of love will soon overtake any concerns.

The third stage of labour

After the birth itself, there is just one final stage of labour, involving the delivery of your placenta. For most women this is not painful, and in the excitement of holding your baby you may not even notice that it has happened.

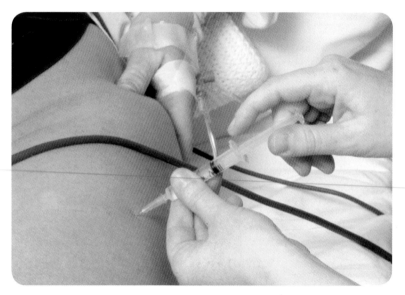

Managed third stage In many cases, your midwife will offer you an injection of a drug known as Syntometrine, which is a combination of Syntocinon (oxytocin), to help the uterus to contract, and Ergometrine, which encourages the uterus to clamp down tightly afterwards.

Post-partum haemorrhage

If the third stage of labour takes longer than about 30 minutes, your risk of heavy bleeding increases slightly.

Primary This occurs when the uterus does not contract down after the birth and is a potentially dangerous condition, causing a drop in blood pressure, rise in pulse rate, and shock.

Secondary If parts of the placenta or membranes are retained, you may experience heavy bleeding and/or infection later. This is quite rare, as the majority of retained placentas are diagnosed and delivered.

Managed or natural third stage?

When your baby is born, the cord is clamped and cut when it has stopped pulsating. In some cases, there may be a slight delay, particularly if you wish to harvest stem cells (see opposite). You can then decide whether you want to have a "managed" or "natural" delivery of your placenta.

Managed An injection of Syntometrine may be offered (see above), which means that you do not have to push to deliver the placenta. There is little blood loss, and a much lower risk of heavy bleeding. It also encourages a speedy third stage, usually lasting five to 15 minutes. However, Ergometrine can cause you to feel nauseous, dizzy, and unwell, and may also cause headaches. For this reason, some hospitals now offer oxytocin on its own, which reduces the side effects.

Natural Some women prefer to deliver the placenta naturally. There can be some accompanying discomfort, and the process can take between 20 and 60 minutes. The average blood loss tends to be higher, although your midwife can administer medication at any stage if she is worried. A natural third stage is not usually recommended if you have had a difficult or long labour or suffered any pregnancy complications.

Stem cell technology

The blood in your baby's umbilical cord is rich with cells known as "stem cells". These have the ability to change into other specific cells and can be used in the treatment of a wide range of conditions.

Stem cells These cells migrate to the bone marrow soon after birth, and transform themselves into various blood-making cells. These are particularly useful in the treatment of health conditions that involve the destruction or malfunction of cells, such as leukaemia, which can potentially be cured by introducing fresh stem cells to the relevant site.

Harvesting You can now harvest and store your baby's cord blood in a blood bank, either to help your baby should he become ill in future, or to aid the treatment of others. Harvesting the cells involves clamping the cord as early as possible, and withdrawing the blood. Some experts are against this practice, as your baby may not get quite as much of this important blood as he might if clamping took place a little later and there was no interruption to the third stage. If you do wish to harvest your baby's stem cells, you'll need to inform your hospital in advance, and find out how you can have the blood collected and stored.

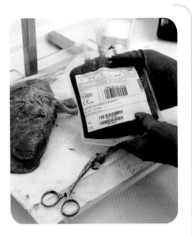

Cells for the future Cord blood for stem cell harvesting can be removed immediately after birth and stored.

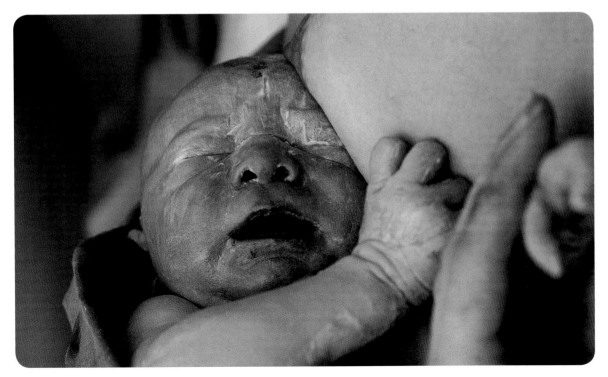

Aiding third stage Holding your baby to the breast will help to encourage the third stage of labour; if you opt to have a managed third stage, you may be largely unaware that your placenta is being delivered as you concentrate on your new baby. This is one reason why many women choose to have this stage managed: to aid delivery of the placenta and membranes, and control bleeding.

A little extra help

No matter how well prepared you are, you may find that your labour is not as straightforward as you had hoped, and some intervention may be required. Try to remain flexible if events lead you into territory you had not anticipated.

Coping with a long labour

Depending on your baby's size and position, strength of contractions, and even the shape of your pelvis, your labour may be longer than expected. Here are some tips to help you cope:

★ Try to relax – fear can interfere with the hormones that keep your labour going strong. Take steps to create the environment you want. If you feel comfortable, you'll find it easier to relax.

★ Eat and drink – even little nibbles of food or sips of something cool and soothing can help to sustain you.

★ Try some aromatherapy oils, either in the bath or in a massage. Lavender will calm and relax, and also help to restore lost energy; frankincense helps to relieve pain, encourage deep breathing, and also rejuvenate.

★ Above all, don't panic! Your midwife will let you know if you reach a point where a little extra help is required.

TOP TIP

In any labour, it is perfectly normal to have periods of intense activity and then rest – try to use quieter moments to catch your breath and even doze a little.

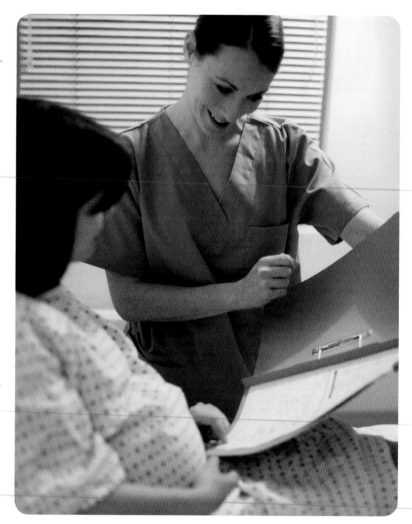

Helping things along If your contractions stop and start or slow down, becoming largely ineffective, your midwife may discuss the possibility of an intravenous drip of Syntocinon to get things going. A long, drawn-out labour can be exhausting for both you and your baby, and it's worth considering options that may help speed things up.

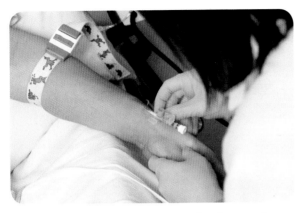

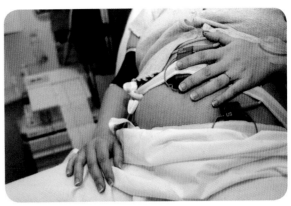

Unproductive labour If your contractions slow down – perhaps because your baby's head is not pressing firmly against your cervix, which signals it to release oxytocin, thereby stimulating contractions – you may want to consider having intravenous oxytocin.

Careful monitoring If you are given intravenous oxytocin, you will be monitored to make sure that contractions do not come on too quickly and are not too strong – paradoxically, oxytocin can lengthen labour if your uterus becomes exhausted by intense over-stimulation.

Breech births

Depending on the position of your breech baby, a vaginal birth may well be possible. You will, however, need to have one-to-one care from a midwife or doctor, to make sure that all proceeds smoothly. You may also have another doctor or nurse present to offer resuscitation, if required.

Before delivery In most cases, you will be aware that your baby is in a breech position before labour and an attempt may be made to turn her (known as external cephalic version or ECV). This is successful in about 50 per cent of cases.

Positioning for a breech birth You will need to adopt a position – perhaps with your feet in stirrups, standing, or on all fours – that allows your midwife or doctor to have access to your baby. Her arms and legs may be manipulated to make the birth easier. Forceps may be required to ease your baby's head out of the birth canal, after her body has been born.

Precautions You may be hooked up to an IV (intravenous) drip in the event that a Caesarean section becomes necessary, but try not to be alarmed. A great many breech babies are delivered naturally, without any complications.

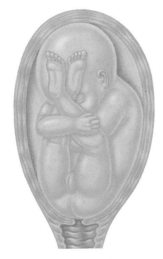

Extended, frank breech This occurs when your baby's bottom is in the downward position, against your cervix. Her hips are flexed, her knees extended, and her feet by her head. A vaginal delivery may be possible.

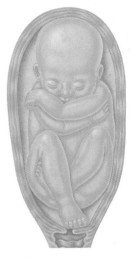

Feet first This is called a "footling breech", and it is unlikely that you'll be able to deliver naturally. If this position has been noted during pregnancy, you will probably have a Caesarean booked.

Caesarean section

A Caesarean section is a surgical procedure that is used to deliver your baby by cutting through your abdominal wall and into the womb. The operation can be done under general anaesthetic, or with a spinal block or epidural, which allows you to remain awake during your baby's birth.

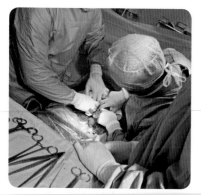

1 **If your Caesarean section** is planned or "elective", you will be offered an epidural anaesthetic or a spinal block. Your partner can usually be present for the operation.

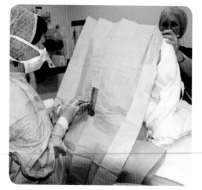

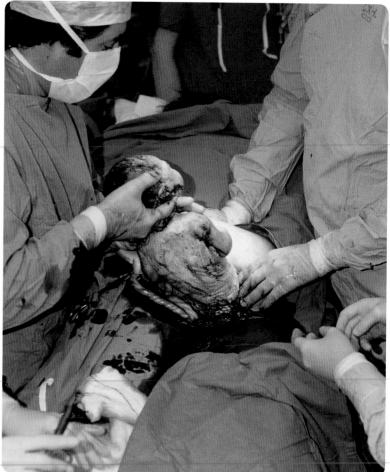

2 **An incision** about 20cm (8in) long is made across your lower abdomen, through the abdominal walls and into the uterus itself. You will be monitored throughout this time, to make sure that your breathing and heartbeat remain stable.

3 **Your baby will be delivered** through the incision – it will take only a few minutes for him to be born. If you are awake, you will feel some tugging and perhaps some pressure, but you will not experience any pain. If you feel discomfort at any stage, the anaesthetist can make adjustments to your pain relief. If you have a general anaesthetic, you will wake up after your baby has been born and your incision has been repaired.

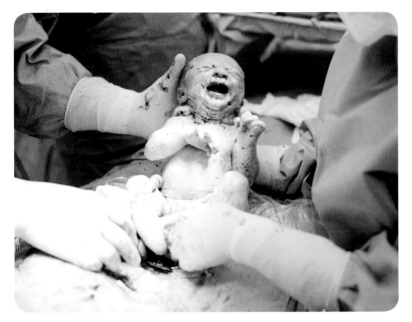

4 **Once your newborn** has been pulled free the cord will be clamped, and then cut. After the placenta has been removed, your surgeon will stitch up the incision in layers, beginning with your womb, then your abdominal muscles, then your skin. Dissolving stitches are usually used, although staples may be used to stitch the skin.

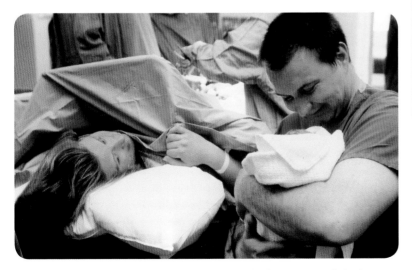

5 **From beginning to end** a Caesarean section takes between 20 and 30 minutes, after which your new baby will be assessed and handed to your partner before undergoing the usual newborn tests (see pp.132–133). It's unlikely that you will be able to hold him until your condition has stabilized. You will be given some pain relief to help you deal with any discomfort that arises when the epidural anaesthetic wears off.

Why a Caesarean?

There are several reasons why a Caesarean section may be indicated, including:

★ A low-lying placenta is covering the exit to the cervix (placenta praevia).
★ Your baby's health is threatened due to lack of oxygen – either before or during labour.
★ The umbilical cord falls forward (cord prolapse), so your baby cannot be delivered easily.
★ There is vaginal bleeding.
★ A long, unproductive labour makes it clear that you are unable to deliver your baby safely on your own.
★ Your baby is in a breech or transverse position (see p.96).
★ You suffer from high blood pressure or other illness.
★ Your baby is too small or too weak to survive a natural birth.
★ Your baby is too big to fit through your pelvis.
★ You are carrying multiple babies (see p.128).

Emergency Caesarean It can be distressing to discover that you need an emergency Caesarean and you'll need the support of your midwife and your birth partner to get you through this experience. You may need an emergency Caesarean if:
★ Your baby's heartbeat shows that he is not coping with contractions; in other words, he becomes distressed.
★ Your cervix stops dilating or dilates too slowly, causing you and your baby to become exhausted.
★ Your placenta begins to come away from the wall of your uterus, posing a risk of haemorrhaging.
★ Your baby doesn't move down into your pelvis, perhaps because he is simply too big for the size of it.

Special deliveries

Every labour is different, and there are various factors or even unexpected events during labour that may mean your baby needs to be delivered with extra assistance – and may need some special care after the birth.

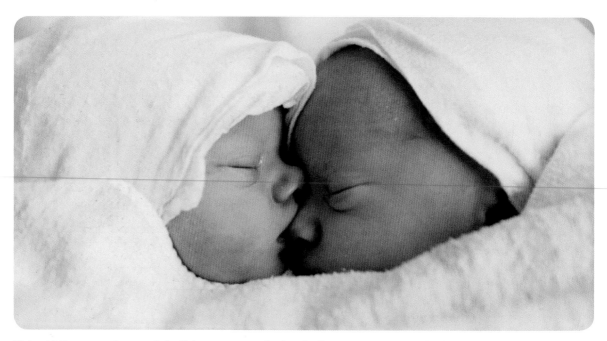

Giving birth to more than one baby Twins or more are often born by Caesarean section a couple of weeks before their official due date. This helps to make sure that you don't go into natural labour, which could pose a threat to the babies' health. If you do decide to try for a vaginal birth, it will be attended by an obstetrician, and you and your babies will be continuously monitored throughout.

Multiple births

Multiple pregnancies are considered high risk, which means that you will receive extra monitoring, and may be advised to have a Caesarean section, depending on the position of your babies and any complications. If you are able to have a vaginal birth, your twins will be delivered one at a time.

Vaginal delivery The delivery of your first baby may require assistance, with a ventouse or forceps, so that your doctor can see to your second baby as quickly as possible. The placenta is usually left in your uterus until your second baby has been born. It's common for second babies to be delivered within an hour of the first. Many twins are smaller than singletons, which makes them easier to deliver.

Special care If your babies are full term, special care may not be required; however, many multiple births occur early, and your babies may require ventilators or incubators until they have sufficiently developed.

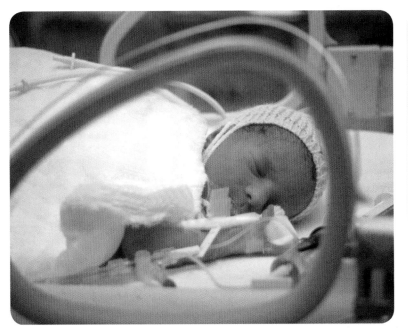

Premature babies Babies born before 37 weeks are classed as premature. Advances in technology mean that premature babies now have a much higher survival rate – even those as young as 22 weeks. Most will need to spend some time in a special care baby unit.

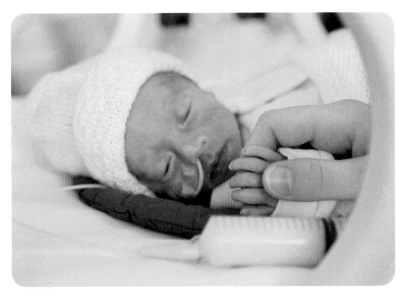

Feeding your special care baby Very tiny babies may need to be fed by syringe. You will be encouraged to express breastmilk, which will be fed to your baby, giving her everything she needs to have the best possible chance of growing and developing well.

Premature labour

Any woman can go into premature labour, and in 40 per cent of cases the causes are unknown.

Possible causes We do know that multiple pregnancies, pre-eclampsia, antenatal haemorrhaging, illnesses (such as diabetes or high blood pressure), cervical incompetence, and abnormalities in your baby can cause you to go into labour before 37 weeks. It's also possible that an infection can trigger early labour.

Onset of labour If contractions start, and become increasingly close together, you may be in labour. If your membranes rupture and you lose amniotic fluid, labour becomes even more likely. Once your cervix begins to dilate, it is too late to stop the labour; however, drugs can be administered to slow it down, which gives your baby a little more time in the womb. Steroids may also be offered to help your baby to breathe.

Complications Babies born after 34 weeks have a much lower risk of complications, as their systems are almost completely mature. Babies under 28 weeks must be delivered in a hospital with a neonatal intensive care unit. Premature babies are at risk of respiratory distress syndrome (problems breathing), hypothermia (they cannot yet regulate their body temperature), low blood sugar, jaundice (see p.134), infection, and eye problems. In many cases, however, your premature baby will be just fine, simply needing plenty of love, care, and attention, as she is assisted during her first days or weeks outside the womb.

Beginning family life

At last, the waiting is over, worries about labour are a thing of the past, and your beautiful baby is lying in your arms. As your recovery gets underway, both you and your partner can start getting to know your new family member.

Your checks

Soon after your baby is delivered, your midwife or doctor will check you over to make sure that all is well.

Postnatal checks Your midwife or doctor will assess your vital signs (pulse and blood pressure), and your uterus will be palpated to check that it is returning to its pre-pregnant state. Your midwife will discuss any pain you are experiencing, and the best ways to manage it. Your perineum will be examined to make sure that tears or episiotomy cuts are starting to heal. Your temperature will be taken and your blood will be checked if you were previously anaemic. If you are Rhesus negative and your baby is Rhesus positive you will be offered an anti-D injection within 72 hours of the birth (see p.57). Your urine may be also tested to check your kidneys are working properly.

Bleeding All women bleed after childbirth, and this blood is known as "lochia". It is, in fact, blood and tissue from the lining of the uterus. At the beginning, it can be quite heavy and red (especially after lying down overnight). It will gradually become pinker and lighter until, around 10 days after the birth, there is just a small amount of white or yellowish discharge. Some women can bleed for up to four weeks.

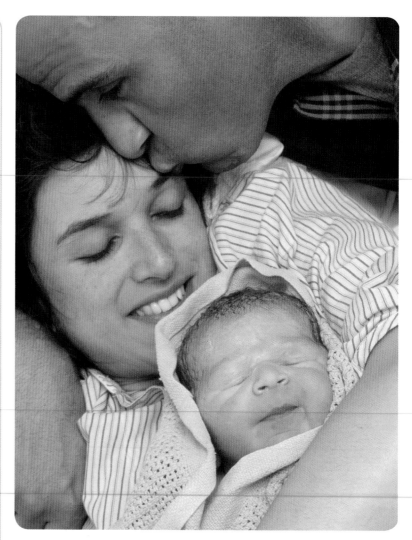

Joint celebration It's natural for dads to feel a little shell-shocked by the process of labour. However, as soon as your baby is born, you can begin your new life together as parents. Take time to celebrate this momentous occasion, and take pride in your wonderful achievement.

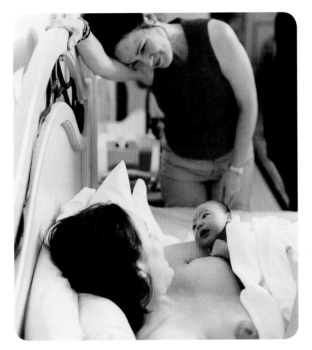

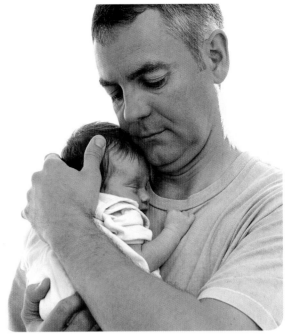

Starting breastfeeding After giving birth, the sooner that you are able to get your baby to your breast – and preferably skin-to-skin – the easier it will be to breastfeed successfully. Holding your baby close will encourage the process of bonding, while breastfeeding can also help your uterus to contract back to its pre-pregnancy size.

Dad's turn Your partner will enjoy his first moments alone with his new son or daughter, and close contact is essential for the bonding process. Having carried your baby for nine months, it's natural to feel a bit nervous about handing him over to anyone, but take advantage of this opportunity to get a little much-needed rest.

Recovering from a Caesarean section

A Caesarean is a major operation, and although you may feel fine immediately after surgery, it's important to take the time to rest and recover.

You will be offered medication to deal with any pain, and this will be chosen and carefully monitored so that you can begin and continue to breastfeed.

Coping with emotions It's normal to feel very tired and tearful – particularly if the Caesarean was not planned – and you may also feel quite shocked. Make sure you take advantage of all the support offered by the professionals in the hospital – if you need more information to understand why a Caesarean was necessary, they'll be able to help.

Breastfeeding You can breastfeed as normal, but may find it more comfortable to place a pillow across your abdomen, to support the weight of your baby. You can also use a pillow to press down on your abdomen when you laugh, cough, or go to the loo, to ease any discomfort.

Avoid lifting Ask your midwife to show you how to roll out of bed and upright, so that you don't need to use your tummy muscles, and ask for your baby to be handed to you, rather than attempting to lift him yourself. You shouldn't lift anything heavier than your baby for the first six weeks after a Caesarean.

Pain relief Afterpains and trapped wind can be more uncomfortable after a Caesarean, so use your breathing exercises to get through them and don't hesitate to accept any pain relief offered.

Accepting help Most importantly, look after yourself. You and your baby must be your first and only priorities until you feel yourself again, and this can take a few weeks. You'll need more rest than mums who have delivered vaginally, so get as much support and help as you can.

After the birth

Having spent nine long months in your womb, your baby will need an assessment to make sure that everything is in working order, and that she is able to breathe on her own. There is a series of tests and checks that are performed on all babies shortly after the birth; they don't take long, however, and you'll soon have your new baby back in your arms.

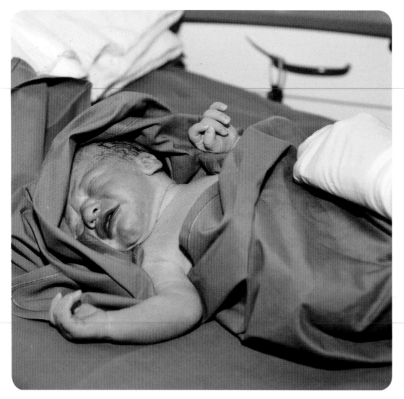

First checks The APGAR test (see opposite) is performed at one and five minutes after the birth, and rates your baby's colour, heart rate, behaviour, activity, and breathing, on a scale of zero to 10. As well as this, your baby will be given a top-to-toe assessment within 48 hours to check for any problems or conditions. This involves examining her head, ears and eyes, mouth, skin, heart, lungs, genitals, hands and feet, spine, hips, and reflexes (see pp.136–37). Most babies pass all of the checks easily, and, in most cases, small problems can be resolved. If there are any concerns, further investigations may be required, but if this is the case try not to worry.

Identifying problems

Your baby may need further tests or monitoring if any potential problems are identified. Common reasons include:

★ A low APGAR score – 6 or below.

★ A low birth weight (see below).

★ Your baby is premature.

★ You had a long delivery and your baby suffered distress.

★ Your waters broke early and you didn't go into established labour for more than 24 hours.

★ Examination shows an abnormality.

★ She is clearly jaundiced (see p.134).

★ She has indiscriminate genitalia.

★ Her breathing or heart rate is faster or slower than expected.

★ She is not a healthy, robust colour.

★ Her muscles and reflexes do not respond as expected.

★ She has a high temperature.

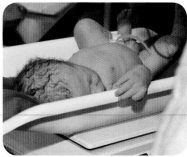

Measurements Your baby will be weighed and measured, and the circumference of her head will be noted. After about 10–14 days you will be given a Personal Child Health Record book to continue to record these measurements and keep tabs on her progress as she develops. Any baby born weighing less than 2.5kg (5lb 8oz) is considered "low birth weight", and will be carefully monitored.

The APGAR score

The Apgar test is undertaken minutes after the birth, and involves watching your baby to check that all is well. Five factors are used to evaluate her condition and each is scored on a scale of 0 to 2. The five scores are added together to calculate the Apgar score. A score of 10 is the highest possible.

APGAR Sign	2	1	0
Appearance (skin colour)	Normal colour all over (hands and feet are pink)	Normal colour (but hands and feet are bluish)	Bluish-grey or pale all over
Pulse (heart rate)	Normal – above 100 beats per minute	Below 100 beats per minute	Absent (no pulse)
Grimace (responsiveness or "reflex irritability")	Pulls away, sneezes, or coughs with stimulation	Facial movements only (grimace) with stimulation	Absent (no response to stimulation)
Activity (muscle tone)	Active, spontaneous movement	Arms and legs flexed with little movement	No movement, "floppy" tone
Respiration (breathing)	Normal rate and effort, good cry	Slow or irregular breathing, weak cry	Absent (no breathing)

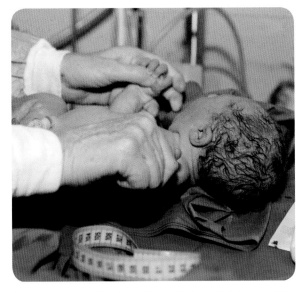

Assessments and jabs Soon after the birth you baby's eyes will be checked for cataracts, infection, or any other problems. Her nasal passages may also be cleared with a suction bulb so that she can breathe more easily, and her temperature taken. With your consent, she'll be given vitamin K by injection or orally, to help her blood clot, and 5–8 days after the birth she'll also be given a heel-prick blood test that tests for enzyme deficiencies and genetic conditions.

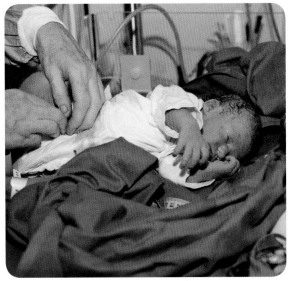

Genital examination Babies frequently have swollen genitals at birth as a result of maternal hormones engorging the tissues (girls sometimes have vaginal discharge for the same reason) but this will settle quickly. Your baby's genitals will be examined to check that they appear normal, and that she is able to urinate. If your baby is a boy, his penis will be looked at to make sure that the opening is at the end, and the doctor will check that his testicles have descended.

Special care babies

If there are any concerns about your baby's health, he may be placed in a special care baby unit (SCBU), where he can be observed and given the treatment he needs. Although this can be upsetting, try to stay calm. Your baby will need you, and he will be getting the best care available.

Why special care?

There are many reasons why your baby may be placed in a special care baby unit.

Premature babies Babies who are born earlier than 34 weeks may need extra help breathing, feeding, and maintaining their body temperature (see p.129). Twins or other multiples will often need assistance after birth, not only because they may be born early but also because they are often much smaller than singleton full-term babies.

Special cases All babies who are very small or have life-threatening conditions – usually affecting their breathing, heart, and circulation – will need some extra attention. Babies born to diabetic mums, or who endured a difficult delivery, may need to be observed for a short period of time. Special care may also be required if your baby is born with marked jaundice – a build up of the pigment bilirubin in the blood (see opposite).

Postnatal surgery Some babies will require surgery shortly after the birth. Your baby may be placed in special care in advance of this, and after any procedures.

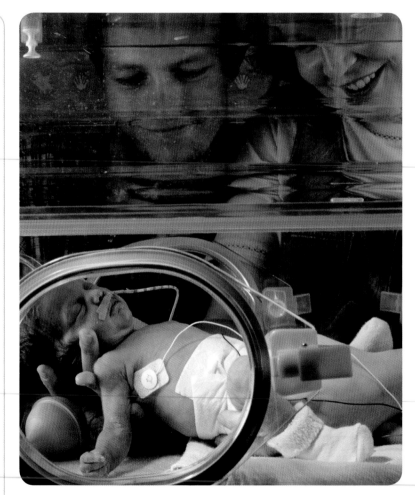

Bond and heal Your special care baby will be placed in an incubator, which can be accessed from openings in the sides. This will allow you to touch, stroke, and even gently hold him. Don't underestimate the importance of this. Not only will it encourage bonding between you and your baby, but it will also help him to heal. The power of touch is well documented, and can greatly enhance your baby's growth, development, and recovery.

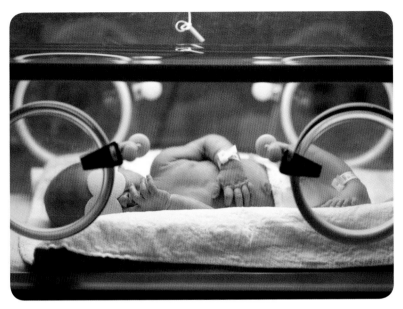

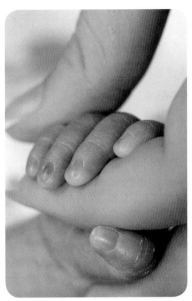

Treatment for jaundice This normally involves placing your baby under a special blue light in a light-box, which looks rather like an incubator, or wrapping him in a light-emitting blanket for a few days. In either case, he will be observed and monitored to make sure that his bilirubin levels are falling and his liver is beginning to do its job. He may also need some help with his fluid intake, to make sure that he gets plenty to drink.

Restricted touch You may only be able to practise "still holding": putting your hand gently on your baby's body for a few seconds. However, the impact of this on his health can be immeasurable.

What your special care baby needs

Your first instinct as a mum or dad will be to hold your baby and try to make things better, and it can come as a shock if physical contact is limited.

You may also be distressed to find that you can't breastfeed your baby, and that he is all on his own in an incubator or specially designed cot.

Your role Try to bear in mind that your role as a parent is as important as ever. Your baby will need to hear your familiar voice, and will feel greatly reassured by your physical presence, even if it is for just a few moments at a time. If possible, you can ask to hold your baby for short periods of time. In some units you'll be encouraged to give "kangaroo care", which means your baby is tucked up against you, feeling your warmth, hearing your heartbeat, and smelling your scent. Special care babies held like this have been shown to gain weight more quickly than those left on their own in their cots or incubators.

Breastfeeding Breastmilk still remains the most important source of nutrition for your baby, and you will be encouraged to express your milk – particularly the extremely nutritious early milk, known as colostrum, which contains valuable nutrients and antibodies that can help your baby to get well. He can take this milk by syringe, tube, cup, or bottle. If you aren't able to produce enough milk yet, your baby may be offered pre-term formula or breastmilk that has been donated to a milk bank at the hospital. Either way, carry on expressing as this will stimulate your breasts to continue making milk to meet his needs.

Talk to the nurses Ask the staff to explain the role of the various pieces of equipment around your baby, and ask them regularly for an update on his condition. It's natural to feel stressed and anxious and the specialist nurses will be only too happy to ease your mind and reassure you that your baby is getting the best possible care.

Speak up for your baby If you are concerned about his care or you aren't sure that a procedure is right for your baby, don't hesitate to follow your instincts and voice your concerns to the doctors and nurses in the unit.

Newborn checks

Within the first 48 hours or so after your baby's birth, a more thorough series of tests will be carried out. If you've had a home birth or you've been discharged soon after the birth, they can be done in your home.

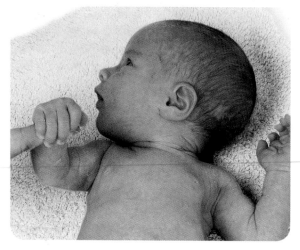

Grasping reflex Your baby will be born with a series of reflexes, which will be checked by your doctor or midwife. The grasping reflex is tested by touching the palm of your baby's hand. Her fingers will curl around and grip your finger or whatever object is used for the test. This reflex is usually in place until she is about six months of age.

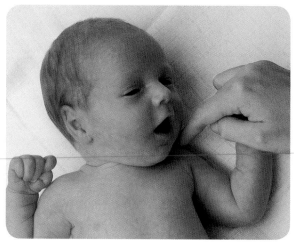

Rooting reflex From birth until about four months of age, this reflex will cause your baby to instinctively turn her face when her cheek is touched. Her mouth will open and she will anticipate being fed. This reflex helps when breastfeeding, as the simple act of pressing her cheek to your breast will encourage her to open her mouth to feed.

Other reflexes

Your baby will be born with a number of other reflexes, which will help her to adjust to life outside the womb and ensure her survival. Sometimes these reflexes are weaker than expected after the birth; however, a long labour or medication given to you during labour can be at the root of the problem.

Moro or startle reflex When your baby's head is allowed to flop backwards she will respond by flinging out her arms, with her fingers outstretched, and stretching her legs. This reflex disappears at about two months of age.

Plantar grasp This occurs when you stroke the sole of your baby's foot. Her toes will spread and her foot will turn slightly inwards. It is normal in children up to two years old, but it disappears as the nervous system develops.

Sucking reflex If you touch the roof of your baby's mouth with your finger, a dummy, or a bottle teat, she will instinctively begin to suck. By about two or three months of age, this reflex will disappear and she will voluntarily suck.

Stepping reflex This involves your baby "walking" well before she is able to do so physically. If you hold her upright and place her feet on a flat surface, she will "walk" by placing one foot in front of the other. It disappears by about four months.

First newborn check

Your baby's first medical checks will take place with you present, and will cause her no discomfort. Your doctor or midwife will explain everything as they review your baby's physical condition, and will point out and discuss with you any potential areas of concern they may find.

Hospital birth If you have given birth in hospital, then you will probably be visited by a paediatrician shortly afterwards. Don't worry that this means there is something wrong, the hospital simply has to establish that all is well before you can both be discharged to go home.

Home birth If you have had a home birth, then the medical checks will probably be carried out in your home by your midwife or GP. In most cases all will be well, but if you're too tired to ask questions, you can do so at your baby's six- to eight-week check (see pp. 182–83).

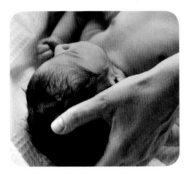

Head This will be examined to make sure the shape is consistent with the birth. It's often moulded or a little squashed. The fontanelle (the soft spot at the top of your baby's head) will also be checked, and any bruising or birthmarks will be noted.

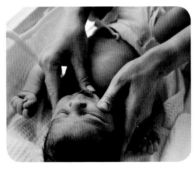

Mouth This will be examined to make sure that the roof of your baby's mouth (palate) is complete, and that her tongue moves freely; if it is too anchored at the bottom of her mouth, she may suffer from "tongue-tie", which restricts normal movement.

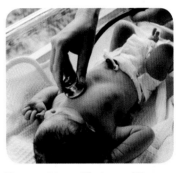

Heart and lungs Her heart will be listened to, to make sure there are no extra sounds or murmurs. She will be checked for a pulse in her groin area (femoral pulse) and her lungs will be checked to be sure they are clear of fluid.

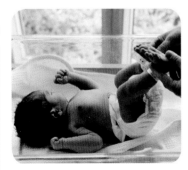

Hands, feet, legs, and arms Fingers and toes will be counted and checked for webbing. Your doctor will also look at the palm creases – if there aren't two on each hand, there is a small chance your baby suffers from Down's syndrome.

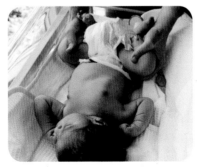

Hips Your baby's hips will be checked to assess the stability of the joints. Her legs will be opened wide and then bent and unbent. "Clicky hips" occur when the hip joint is too loose and the thighbone dislocates itself and will need further investigations.

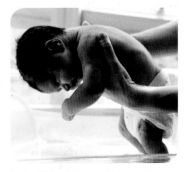

Spine This will be checked to make sure that it is straight, and any dimple at the base of her spine – known as a sacral dimple – will be examined. A very deep sacral dimple can indicate a problem with the lower part of her spinal cord.

Getting started

Once your baby has been given a clean bill of health, the real fun begins. You will now be able to take charge of his care, bathing him, feeding him, dressing him, and settling him down to sleep. The first few days can be daunting, but you'll soon settle into a routine, and begin to parent with confidence.

TOP TIP

Whispering "shhhh" in your baby's ear and rocking him gently will help mimic the conditions he experienced in the womb and soothe him instantly.

Skin-to-skin contact

There is now strong evidence pointing to the benefits of skin-to-skin contact between mother and baby, and indeed between dads and babies, too.

Research One review of 17 studies found that early skin-to-skin contact between mum and baby improved the success rate of breastfeeding – as well as its duration – and helped to maintain a normal temperature in your baby, encourage stable blood sugar, reduce crying, and improve the process of bonding. One study found that premature babies who were held in skin-to-skin contact had greater head growth than babies held in a traditional way. What's more, the overall physical and emotional health of mums is believed to be positively affected with skin-to-skin contact.

Boosting breastfeeding If your new baby hasn't been placed directly on your chest after birth, remove his babygro and vest and try your first breastfeed "naked".

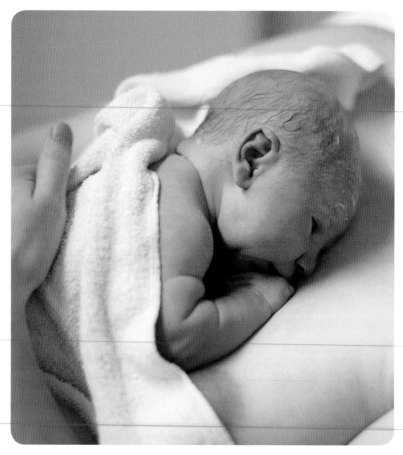

Learning to breastfeed Babies are not born knowing exactly how to breastfeed, although they do have a "rooting reflex" (see p.136). Most babies instinctively "root" within the first hour of being born. Placing your baby on your chest, with your skin against his, will stimulate this reflex, and he will move his head towards the stimulus and open his mouth in search of food.

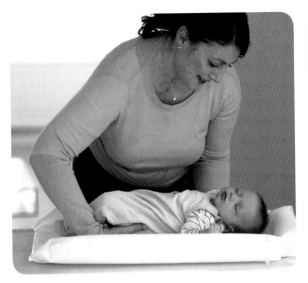

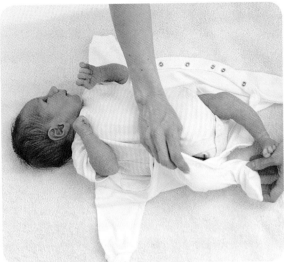

Changing nappies Many babies don't like having their nappies changed, perhaps due to the temporary loss of close contact with mum or dad, and also because it can make them feel cold and uncomfortable. Organize a changing station well in advance to make things as efficient and comfortable as possible.

Dressing your baby In the early days, your baby will not need a vast wardrobe of clothes. He'll be most comfortable in a light cotton all-in-one, with poppers that allow you easy access for changes. Place him on a firm surface and lay out his babygro. Gently ease his legs in first before guiding his arms into the sleeves.

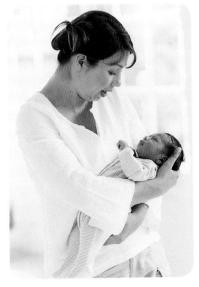

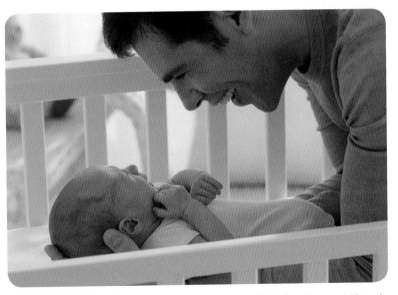

Support his head Your baby's neck muscles will not be fully developed for many months, so when you pick him up, always keep a hand or your arm firmly behind his head, and cradle the length of his body.

Get dad involved It's a great idea to share the care of your baby from the outset. Not only will this give both you and dad a chance to relax and rest, but also your baby will soon become accustomed to being settled by both of you. This can be invaluable in the middle of the night. It's natural to offer the comfort of a feed when your baby is crying, but in some cases, he just wants to be held or settled down to sleep.

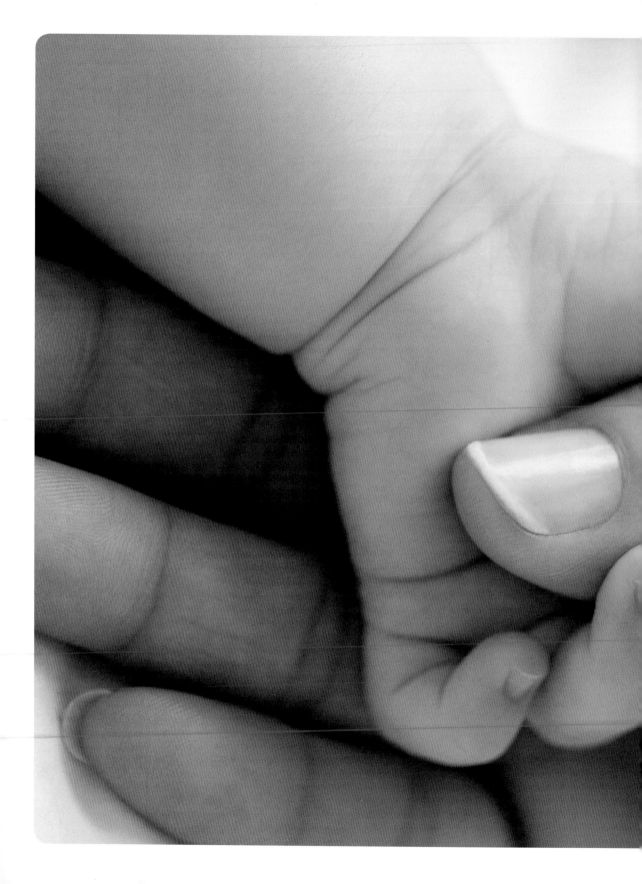

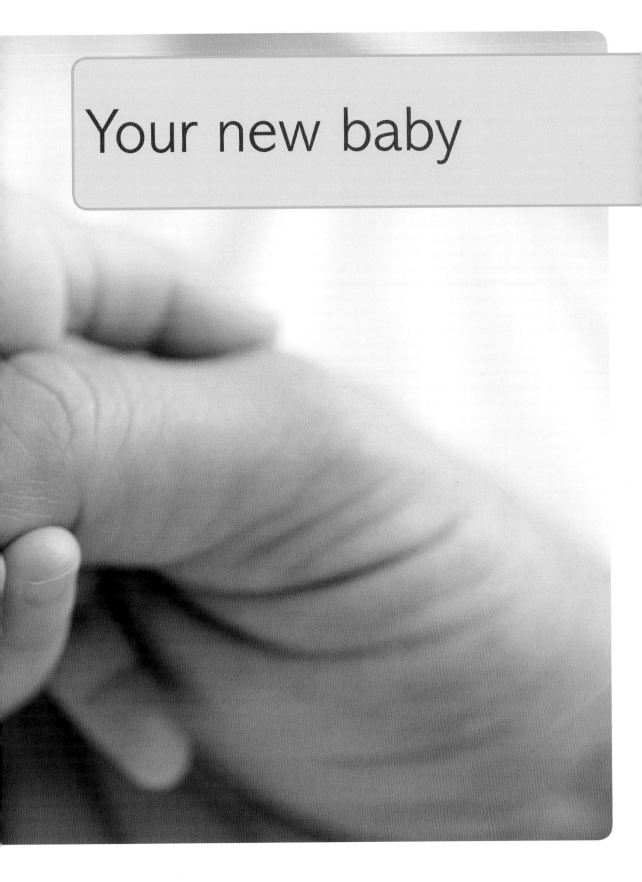

Your new baby

YOUR NEW ARRIVAL

As soon as you arrive home with your new baby, the process of parenting can truly begin. She will undoubtedly have her own temperament from the outset, and it may take time to get to know what she wants and needs. The most important thing you can do is to relax and enjoy spending time with her.

KEEPING HER COMFORTABLE

All babies cry when they are not comfortable, and you may be unnerved if it's unclear why your baby's distressed. Most of the time a feed, a clean nappy, some close comfort with mum or dad, a warm place to sleep, and a little stimulation will keep her calm and content. What she needs most of all, however, is your love and affection. She'll soon begin to trust you, and feel safe and confident to grow, develop, and eventually explore the world around her.

GROWING IN CONFIDENCE

As you learn to recognize and deal with your baby's cries, and get to grips with the basics of babycare, you'll soon settle into a gentle routine. No two babies are the same, and no technique will always work, but if you have a clear idea of the best way to go about bathing and changing her, making sure that she is well fed and putting on weight, caring for her when she is ill or distressed, and keeping her stimulated and comforted according to her individual needs, the rest will fall into place. Share your concerns with your partner and your midwife, doctor, or health visitor. There are wonderful systems in place to make sure that new mums and dads get the support and guidance they need to parent confidently.

GETTING ORGANIZED

As you and your baby get to know one another, you'll soon begin to recognize some patterns emerging; she may be sleepy at roughly the same times, and want to settle down for the night after a good, early-evening feed. She may be alert for an hour or so in the afternoons or early morning, and enjoy a little gentle play. Knowing roughly what to expect and when can make your life immeasurably easier. However, it is important to resist the temptation to get on with housework or anything else that doesn't absolutely need to be done. Instead, spend your time resting and organizing things so that daily life with

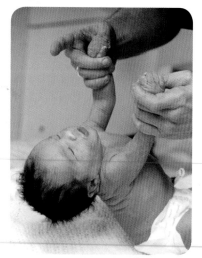

Gaining head control About six to eight weeks after she is born, your doctor will give your baby a thorough postnatal check to make sure she is thriving and that her development is progressing as it should.

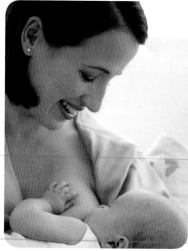

Breastfeeding It is well-documented that breastfeeding offers your baby significant long-term health benefits, so persevere – it is a skill that once learnt can be undertaken at any time and in any place.

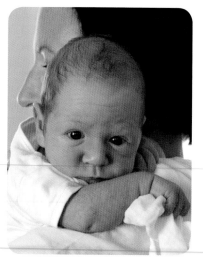

Little personality Every baby is different, and right from the start your newborn will demonstrate that she already has her own personality. Getting to know her in the early weeks can be exciting and rewarding.

your baby can be smoother and more efficient. For example, take a moment to organize yourself and your baby's belongings – topping up the changing stations or the changing bag with nappies and fresh flannels, laying out her towel and pyjamas in advance of the bath, and making sure that you have a nutritious snack and plenty to drink when you settle down to feed your baby – can help you to keep on top of things, and give you more time to relax and enjoy being a new parent.

LOOKING AFTER YOURSELF

There is no doubt that a new baby can be exhausting, and you may find yourself at the end of your tether from time to time. Try to remember that you are not alone. Work on your relationship with your partner, and work out a system for taking care of your baby, your household, and yourselves with the minimum of fuss. Make sure you take the time to relax, eat well, get outside into the fresh air, and see friends and family who will lift your spirits and provide you with the support you need. The weeks to come will be full of "firsts", as you establish breastfeeding and learn to care for and comfort your baby – make sure you make time for yourself as you adapt to all the changes that come with parenthood.

ABOVE ALL, ENJOY!

Babies grow and develop dramatically in the first weeks and months of life, and it won't be long before your tiny baby is mobile, and beginning to show the first signs of independence. The early days are precious, and absolutely critical to your baby's emotional and physical health, so take the time to settle in. Gaze in wonder at the little being you've created, and revel in the comfort and warmth of feeding and holding her. No matter what you did before you became pregnant, or how organized or efficient you may be, it's important to remember that your top priority – and your most important job – is now caring for your new baby. This involves keeping her safe, happy, and comfortable, no matter how long that takes. You've done something truly amazing, so pat yourself on the back, sit back, and enjoy.

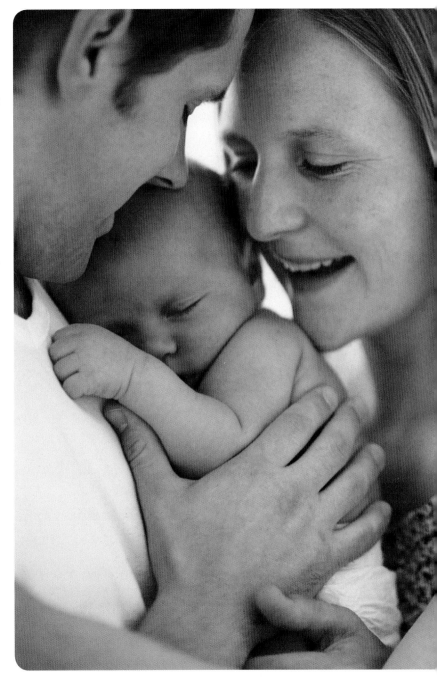

Enjoy family time Starting a family together is an exciting time for any couple, and by supporting each other and working together as you get to grips with the highs and lows of parenthood, you can make your relationship stronger than ever.

The first few days

Your days will quickly become full of "firsts" as you get to grips with bathing, changing, and feeding your baby, and settle into life as a family. Relax and let the joy of new parenthood see you through the wonderful weeks to come.

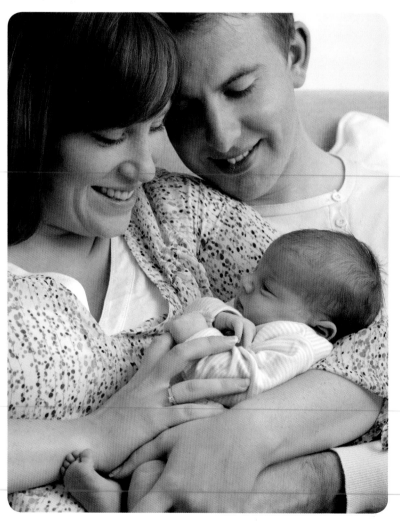

Baby blues

At least seven out of 10 women experience the phenomenon known as "baby blues".

Early days About three or four days after your baby is born, you may feel weepy, overwhelmed, tired, and low. This is completely normal and is due to the huge hormonal shifts that take place after giving birth, as well as the fact that caring for a new baby is unbelievably tiring. The most important thing is to get help and support from your partner, your family, and the health professionals who are there to help you.

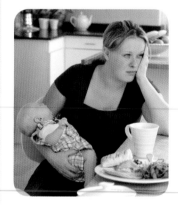

Postnatal depression If symptoms don't pass within two weeks, talk to your doctor or midwife as you may be suffering from postnatal depression.

Getting to know each other Your baby will love being close to you, and will revel in your familiar smell, voice, and touch. After being tightly nestled in your womb for so many months, he'll feel most secure being firmly held in your arms. The more time you spend with your baby, the easier the process of bonding will be, and the closer your relationship.

Coping with twins

Here are some tips to make things easier in the early days of parenting twins:

★ Place your babies down together to sleep; they are more likely to find comfort when they are in close proximity to each other than they are to wake one another up.

★ Get some help for at least two or three weeks, until you've worked out a routine. Try to organize things so that you have help at crucial times, such as bathtime and bedtime.

★ Forget about the housework – something has to give.

★ Don't panic. It can be difficult to manage holding two babies, let alone comforting or feeding them at the same time – you'll soon acquire the necessary juggling skills.

★ Run a tight ship. Set out a babygro and towels for the bath whenever you get a second; throw in a load of laundry while you are warming a bottle; and spend a few moments online getting a preset grocery list delivered. You'll feel more in control when some of the basics are in place.

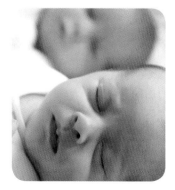

Take your time You'll soon adapt to meeting the demands of your babies, but allow yourself time to get there.

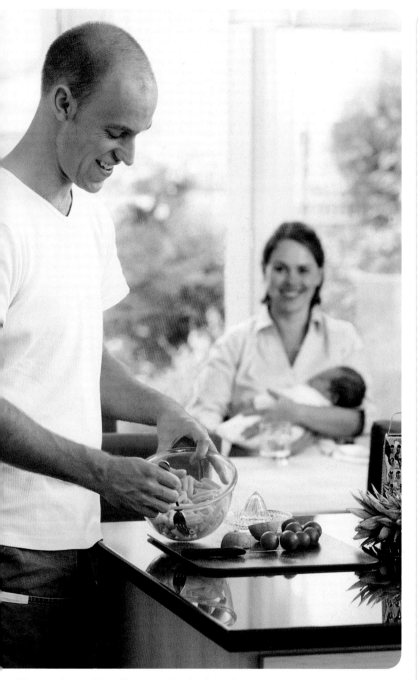

Sharing the workload New parenthood is definitely a time for sharing household responsibilities, and you may have to rethink the division of labour. Providing support for one another can make your relationship with your partner that much stronger.

145

Looking after yourself

Try to remember that newborn babies have very basic needs – as long as they are fed, comforted, and clean, you can safely rest and allow your body to recover.

Easing discomfort

Giving birth can be an uncomfortable business, and after poor sleep in the latter weeks of pregnancy, an exhausting labour, and perhaps some stitching, medication, or other interventions, you may be feeling a little battered. Here are some ways to help ease the discomfort:

★ If you've had stitching, buy a blow-up ring to sit on. This avoids placing any pressure on your perineum.

★ Add a drop or two of lavender oil to your bathwater This will encourage healing and ease any itching.

★ A cool gel pack on the area can ease discomfort and reduce swelling.

★ Pouring a jug of cool water over your vagina as you urinate can be soothing.

★ Take some paracetamol or use your breathing exercises to get through any after-pains as your uterus contracts back to its pre-pregnancy size.

★ If you are nervous about – or having difficulty with – bowel movements, make sure you increase your intake of fibre, and drink plenty of fresh water. If you are still struggling, ask your doctor for a mild laxative to move things along.

★ A little gentle exercise should help you to relax enough to sleep well.

★ Exhaustion goes with the territory, so try to sleep when your baby sleeps.

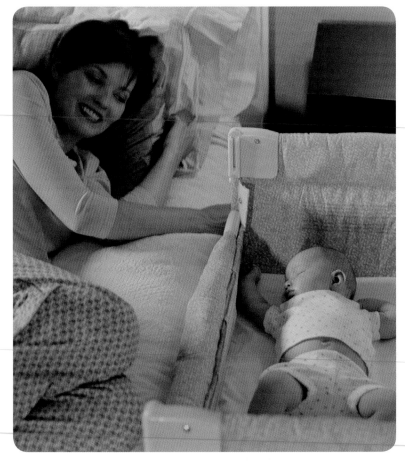

Avoid placing pressure on yourself There is no reason why a new mum has to be superwoman. Let the housework go for a while, and take advantage of periods when your baby is sleeping. The current guidance is to keep your baby in the same room as you for the first few months, so curl up next to her, put your feet up, and get a little sleep.

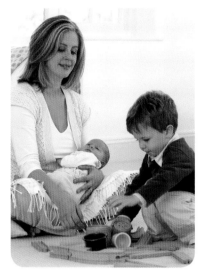

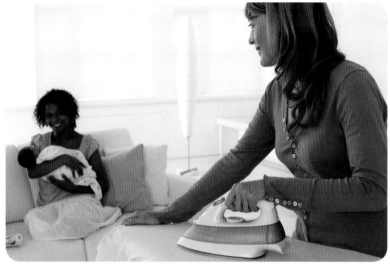

Older children Your routine will change a little as you adapt to life with a new baby, but simply spending time with your other, older children will reassure them. A special gift for them "from" the baby can also help.

Accept help Don't hesitate to take up offers of help from friends or family. A new baby can be hard work, and your body will need some time to recover after the birth. What's more, breastfeeding can be a fairly time-consuming occupation in the early days, and you'll need all of your resources to keep things going. Put your feet up, enjoy a chat, and make yourself comfortable. A happy, relaxed mum makes a much more confident parent.

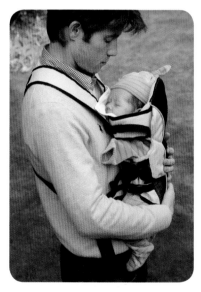

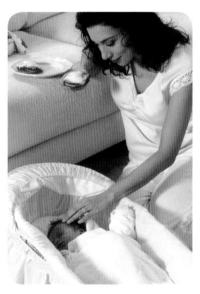

After a Caesarean

There are a few things you can do to speed up recovery after a Caesarean and reduce the risk of complications.

★ Support your womb with your hand or a pillow when you cough, sneeze, and urinate.

★ Breathe deeply to prevent a chest infection – it's very common to breathe too shallowly after surgery because you are fearful of any pain.

★ Move your ankles often, and stay as mobile as you can, to prevent clots from forming in the veins in your legs.

★ Wear over-sized underwear that will not put any pressure on your scar, and keep the area clean with regular, warm showers.

Time to explore There's no reason why your baby can't enjoy her first visit to the great outdoors soon after her birth. Wrap her up warmly, and encourage dad to take her for a walk to give you a little break.

Eat well It may seem difficult to squeeze in time for meals, but eating little and often, and staying hydrated is not just important to keep up your energy levels, but it can also help to prevent postnatal depression.

Baby basics

You may be astonished by the amount of time it can take to care for such a tiny baby – try to remember that no day will ever be perfect and the best approach is to let your baby dictate the proceedings for the first few weeks.

Moving towards a routine

★ **Forget about routines** for the first few weeks. You'll need time to bond, and your baby's routine will eventually assert itself.

★ **Once you know** what your baby likes, and when, you can start to build a routine from there.

★ **Use a schedule** as a guideline, and don't force it. All babies have fussy days, and on other days you may have activities or appointments that mean you are in a different place come nap- or bathtime.

★ **Flexibility is fine,** as long as you do things in roughly the same order, and lead up to bedtime with much the same sequence of events.

★ **There is no reason** why you can't feed on demand while working out a routine, but settling in a familiar chair, with his usual blanket to hand, can lead your baby to associate these things with feeding, and anticipate it.

★ **Offer feeds** at the times that work best for you, and your baby will eventually feed more during these times, and fall into more habitual behaviour.

★ **Take a walk** at roughly the same time each day, then build in a routine for playtime, reading or singing, and his bath.

★ **Try bathing,** reading a story, and then feeding him before putting him down in his bed. Say good night, and leave him, but you must return if he cries. If you do this every night, he will soon begin to see it as a natural event.

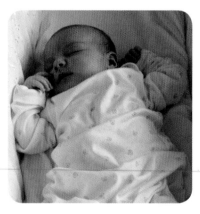

Bedtime Babies should be placed down to sleep on their backs, with their feet at the foot of their cot or basket. It's a good idea to layer blankets, rather than using anything heavy that may cause your baby to overheat.

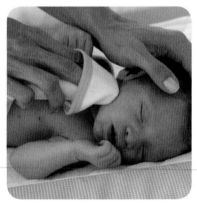

Easy washing Topping and tailing (see p.161) is a good alternative to daily bathing, but if you are pressed for time, or your baby has settled into a restful sleep, a quick wash with a warm flannel will also do the job.

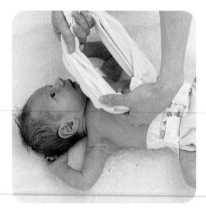

Dressing Many babies aren't happy about being dressed or undressed, so make the proceedings fun. Laugh, smile, pull faces, chat, and sing to your baby, and he'll soon come to enjoy these regular sessions.

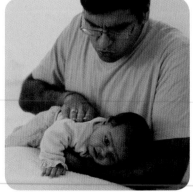

Winding This is an important skill to acquire, as all babies can suffer discomfort from trapped wind. Experiment with different positions to work out the best way to help your baby to release the air bubbles.

Dad's involvement

It can be difficult for some mums to relinquish control in the early days. Mums tend to be most attuned to the needs of new babies, having carried them for nine months and being largely responsible for their nourishment and comfort. It's not surprising that dads can feel left out.

Teamwork Try to remember that your partner may be feeling equally unsettled after the labour, and struggling with the demands of a new baby. He may also be a little jealous that your close relationship has changed, and that your new priority is someone else. It's worth considering that the best parents are those who work as a team, sharing the responsibilities as well as the joys and pleasures of caring for a completely dependent child. Dads also need to be allowed time to bond with their babies, and to establish their own personal relationship.

Share the load As hard as it may seem, try to share the load a little. Let your partner pick your baby up when he wakes, tend to him when he's distressed, change and bathe him, and take him for some "daddy-time" walks. That doesn't mean shift work – it simply involves relaxing a little and letting your partner become and feel involved. Let him enjoy a bath with your baby, or spend some time with him when he wakes early in the morning. Allow your partner to establish his own routine, and make sure you respect and appreciate his efforts and approach. By getting involved, your partner will also understand some of the difficulties you are experiencing and be able to support you more. You have many years of shared parenting ahead, and working together from the beginning will make it all much easier in years to come.

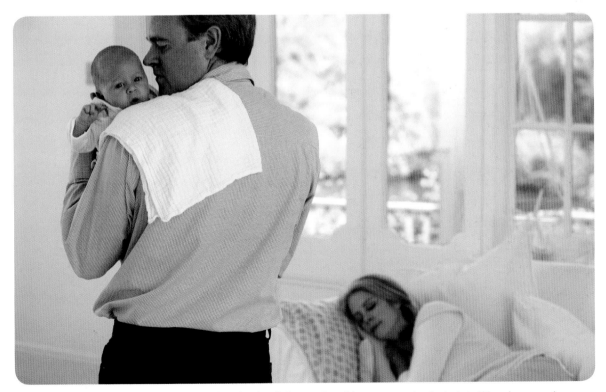

Taking turns It doesn't take two parents to soothe a fractious baby, or to keep him company when he is alert. Although you may be fascinated by your baby's activities, or feel distressed and want to be with him when he is upset, it's a good idea to take it in turns to care for him from time to time, so that you both build your relationship with him and also to allow both of you to get some much-needed rest.

Breastfeeding

We know that breast milk provides the best possible nutrition for your baby, but breastfeeding itself can be a bit of an art. However, with guidance and perseverance, you'll soon find it the best and easiest way to feed your baby.

Breast is natural

Even if you can only manage it for a few weeks or months, breastfeeding is undoubtedly the best choice for your baby.

Health benefits The composition of breastmilk changes constantly, to allow for your baby's individual growth and changing nutritional needs. Research has found that breastfed babies have fewer incidences of vomiting and diarrhoea, colic, and chronic constipation, and that it protects against gastroenteritis, ear infections, respiratory illnesses, pneumonia, bronchitis, kidney infections, and septicaemia (blood poisoning). There is also a reduced risk of childhood diabetes in breastfed babies, as well as protection against allergies, asthma, and eczema.

Fat The fat contained in human milk is more digestible for babies than cow's milk and allows for greater absorption of fat-soluble vitamins into the bloodstream from the baby's intestine. This is important because healthy fats are necessary for optimum growth and development, particularly in the brain.

SIDS There is a reduced risk of sudden infant death syndrome – in particular, research has found that of every 87 deaths from SIDS, only three took place in breastfed babies.

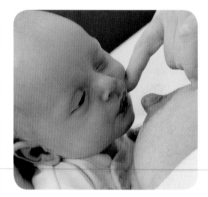

1 **Gently stroking** your baby's cheek or the corner of her mouth will stimulate her rooting reflex, and she will open her mouth to seek out food. The next most important step is to check that she is correctly latched on to your breast.

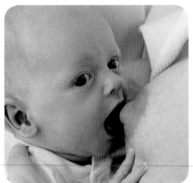

2 **When your baby** opens her mouth wide, bring her to your breast. Her tongue should be down and forward, and your nipple should be aimed at the roof of her mouth. All of the nipple and some of the breast tissue should be in her mouth.

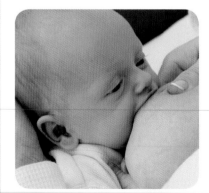

3 **Your baby is correctly positioned** if her tummy is to yours – tummy-to-tummy. Her lower lip will be rolled out and her chin will be against your breast. Her nose should be free of your breast so that she can breathe comfortably.

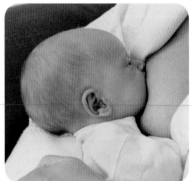

4 **If your baby is properly** latched on, you should hear only a low-pitched swallowing noise – not a sucking or smacking noise – and you should see her jaw moving, a sign that a successful feeding is taking place.

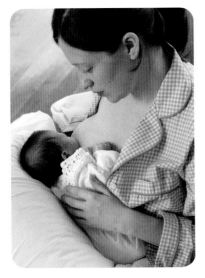

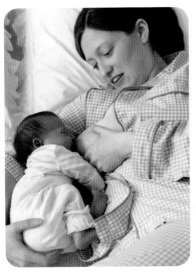

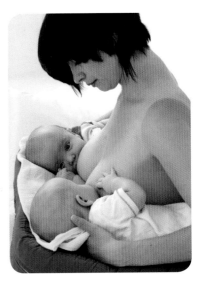

Cradle hold You may wish to experiment with positions to find one that is most comfortable for you. The cradle hold is popular with many mums because latching on is that much easier; you can prop your baby up on a cushion if it's easier to get her directly on to your breast.

Lying down It is possible to feed your baby lying down, and this can be a useful technique if you are experiencing any abdominal discomfort – and for feeding at night. Make sure your baby's tummy is pressed up against yours, and that she has the whole of your nipple in her mouth.

Twins There are several holds for feeding twins simultaneously. Many women enjoy the "rugby" hold, which keeps your babies well supported and allows you to see what they are both doing. It can take some getting used to, but it is by far the most efficient way of getting both babies fed at once.

Winding your baby

Winding prevents your baby from getting air trapped in her digestive system, which can make her uncomfortable, and also prevents her from bringing up all her feed when an air bubble eventually emerges.

Bottle-fed babies All babies need to be winded after a feed – and sometimes even throughout; however, bottle-fed babies do tend to require special attention, as the action of sucking from a bottle rather than the breast means that they take in more air than breastfed babies.

Be prepared To wind your baby, hold her over your shoulder and support her head. Gently rub her back until she makes a suitable expulsion. It's common for some babies to bring up a little milk when they burp (posseting), so make sure you protect your clothes with a muslin or a towel over your shoulder when winding.

Crying Many babies will cry when they have trapped wind, which can interrupt a feed as well as sleep. It is, therefore, always worth winding a crying baby to ascertain if this is the problem. If you have a "windy" baby on your hands, you may need to wind frequently throughout feeds to make sure that she is comfortable enough to feed properly.

Horizontal hold Some babies like to be held horizontally, with their tummies and chests resting across the inside of your forearm, and their heads in the palm of your hand. Keep your baby slightly upright so that air bubbles can be released easily.

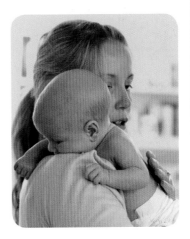

Winding It's sometimes possible to feel an air bubble working its way up your baby's body and out as you rub her back.

Breastfeeding problems

It is absolutely normal for your breasts to feel sore and tender for the first few days. If problems arise, use these tried-and-tested tips to get back on track.

Treating sore, chapped nipples

★ Try to relax when you are feeding, as this will help the milk come more easily.

★ Make sure you get the latch correct; if your baby is feeding with the whole of your nipple and some of the breast tissue in his mouth, you shouldn't experience anything more than a little short-term tenderness.

★ Start feeds on the breast that is the least sore, and when your baby is finished feeding strongly, remove him and feed on the sore breast. If necessary, just express milk from the sore breast until the nipple recovers a little.

★ Try to avoid pulling your baby off your breast, as the suction created by his mouth as he feeds can make it more painful (see right).

★ At the end of a feed, express a little of the rich, fatty milk and rub it over your nipple to encourage healing.

★ Between feeds, keep your bra and T-shirt off for short periods to allow the air to get to your nipples.

★ Avoid using plastic-backed breastpads, and change any pads that become even a little damp.

★ There are some good emollient creams on the market for sore nipples, many of which contain all-natural ingredients, such as chamomile.

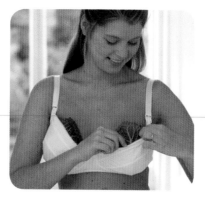

Soothing When you are engorged or suffering from mastitis, try placing cold gel soothers or cabbage leaves in your bra; the enzymes seem to reduce inflammation.

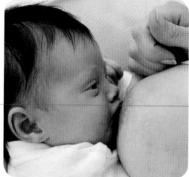

Break the suction If your baby falls asleep or you wish to change breasts, carefully insert your clean little finger into the corner of his mouth so you can pull him away comfortably.

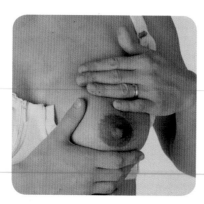

Express to relieve Help to ease engorged breasts by massaging towards your nipple to express a little milk. This is also useful if you are suffering from blocked ducts or mastitis.

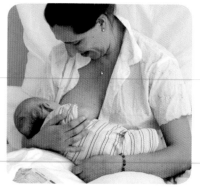

Empty each breast Try to empty one breast before moving on to the next to make sure that your baby gets the hydrating foremilk and the more nutrient-dense hindmilk.

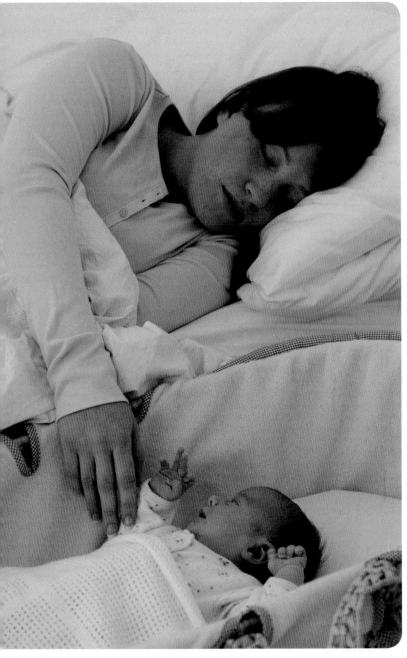

Get some rest Breastfeeding can be exhausting, particularly when you are waking frequently in the night to meet your baby's needs. Try to rest whenever you can, and keep night feeds quiet and efficient. Keep the lighting low at night and once he is fed, wind him, and return him to bed with the minimum of fuss so you can get more rest.

Maintaining your energy levels

Breastfeeding and the physical recovery from labour and delivery can leave you tired and hungry, so it's important to top up your energy levels with healthy snacks throughout the day.

Omega 3 Make sure that you are getting some omega 3 oils, found in fish, nuts, and seeds, in your daily diet; studies have found that these are great for enhancing brain function and keeping depression at bay.

Protein Eat plenty of good-quality protein, which is necessary for your body to produce the neurotransmitter serotonin, which has a calming effect. Scrambled eggs, slices of lean meat, cheese and biscuits, or a little yogurt with fruit all make ideal snacks, as do a handful of nuts or even a tin of baked beans on toast.

Fluids Always keep a drink at your side when breastfeeding. Herbal teas can be iced, and drunk with honey and lemon to refresh. Try chamomile to relax, peppermint to refresh, and rosehip for energy-boosting iron. Fresh water is even better, and a tall glass of fresh juice will give you a much-needed fruit portion, rich in vitamins and minerals. Fatigue and anxiety are symptoms of even moderate dehydration.

Empty calories Avoid sugary and refined snacks, such as crisps, sweet biscuits, and cakes; they may satisfy you in the short term, but your blood-sugar levels will soon plummet leaving you tired and irritable.

Bottle-feeding

There have been a huge number of improvements to formula milk over the last decade, so if you are unable to breastfeed, or simply don't like the idea, it is perfectly possible to raise a healthy, happy baby on formula milk.

Making up a feed

It is essential that you follow the manufacturer's instructions to the letter. Too much of the formula powder or liquid can cause your baby to become constipated, or thirsty; too little may mean that she isn't getting what she needs in terms of nutrition. Many mums choose to use ready-prepared formula, which will be perfectly balanced.

★ Measure the formula carefully. If you are using a scoop, use a clean, sterilized knife to level the powder before tipping it into the bottle of water. Place the teat and cap (or the lid) on the bottle and check that it is secure.

★ Always measure the water into the bottle first and then add the formula powder or concentrated liquid. Shake carefully to make sure that it is well-blended, and that it hasn't clogged the teat.

★ Use cooled, previously boiled water, not mineral water, which will upset the balance of nutrients in the formula.

★ Your newborn will probably take 60–120ml (2–4oz) per feed during her first few weeks, and will most likely be hungry every two to four hours, so will need about six to seven feeds in 24 hours. In general, offer about 150ml of milk per kilogram of body weight (or 2½–3oz per pound) during each 24-hour period until about four or five months of age. If your baby still seems hungry, try offering an extra ounce or two during each feed, to see if that makes a difference.

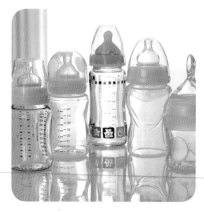

Bottles and teats There is a wide range available, and you can buy anything from anti-colic bottles and those that self-sterilize to "natural" and slow- or fast-flow teats. Try several to see what works best for your baby.

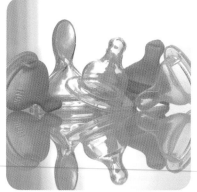

Which teat? Teats should be slow-flowing for new babies, and gradually become "faster" as they get older. Silicone teats are more durable; however, latex tends to be closer to the sensation of a nipple.

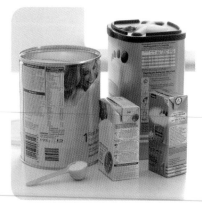

Choosing formula Opt for formula that is appropriate for your baby's age. Most formulas contain roughly the same beneficial ingredients. You can make up formula, or you can buy ready-made.

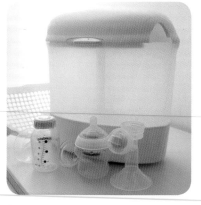

Sterilizing One of the most important pieces of equipment will be your sterilizer. Everything used to make up feeds, as well as the bottles, teats, and caps, will need to be carefully cleaned and sterilized before use.

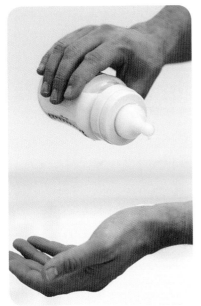

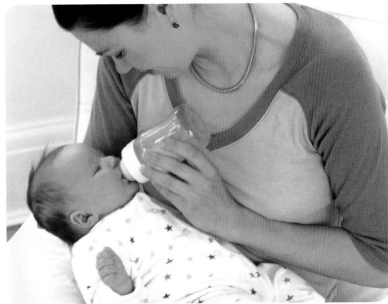

Temperature Always shake the bottle well after heating and test the temperature of your baby's milk on the inside of your wrist before offering her a bottle. It should feel "just warm" to the touch.

Giving a bottle Cradle your baby in a semi-upright position, supporting her head. Don't feed her lying down as formula can flow into the sinuses or middle ear, causing an infection. To prevent your baby from swallowing air as she sucks, tilt the bottle so that the formula fills the neck of the bottle and covers the nipple. If your baby dozes off during her feed she may have wind, which is making her feel full. Sit her up and wind her, then offer some more milk.

Bottle-feeding hygiene

Always make up bottles of formula as and when you need them. In the past, it was common practice to make up a whole raft of bottles, store them in the fridge, and use them as required; however, we now know that this can cause gastroenteritis and other tummy upsets.

Stored bottles Occasionally it just isn't possible to make up bottles on demand. If this is the case, store prepared bottles in the fridge at below 5°C (41°F) for no longer than 24 hours – and less for very young babies. Prepared bottles are best kept in the back of the fridge and not in the door. The temperature of the fridge should be checked regularly.

Warming bottles Warm your baby's bottles using a bottle-warmer or by placing them in a container of hot water; don't leave a bottle warming for more than 15 minutes.

Warm milk Never keep feeds warm as bacteria can grow very quickly in milk. When your baby has finished feeding, always throw away any leftovers.

On the move If you are out and about, place boiling water in a sealed vacuum flask and use this to make up fresh formula when required. Formula liquid or powder should be transported in a sealed, sterile container. You may find it easier to purchase ready-made formula when you plan to be out for long periods of time. It will remain sterile until it's opened, and can be heated as required.

Cold bag storage If necessary, you can make up a bottle or two of formula in advance and, when they are cool, put them in a cold bag containing an ice block. Feeds stored in a cold bag should be used with four hours.

Making up feeds Although it can be tempting to use bottled water when you are away from the house, it is not appropriate for babies. Not only does it contain high levels of minerals (including salt) that your baby doesn't need, but it may also contain bacteria that could make your baby ill.

Disposable nappies

Many parents use disposables at least some of the time, but bearing in mind the environmental impact, it is worth choosing brands that are eco-friendly.

Eco-friendly disposables

From birth to potty training, your baby will use approximately 5,000 disposable nappies, so it's worth trying to reduce their environmental impact. Look for:

★ Nappies made with at least 50 per cent biodegradable materials.

★ Disposables without bleaching agents – a major source of pollution during manufacture and decomposition.

★ Fragrance-, dye-, and latex-free nappies, as these contain fewer harmful waste products (and are kinder to your baby's sensitive skin).

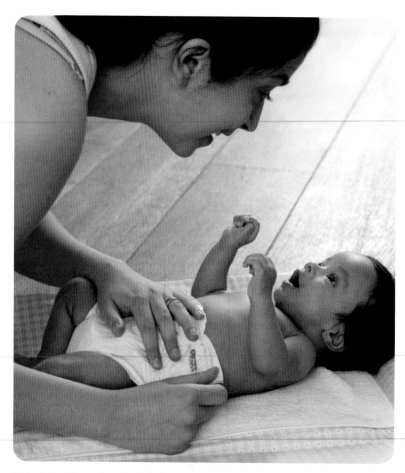

Make it fun Nappy changing isn't always enjoyable for your baby, but engaging him with eye contact, singing, and chatter can help to make it easier. Always take time to clean your baby's bottom properly, wiping from front to back, cleaning all the crevices carefully, and using warm, soapy water or water-based wipes to remove any traces of urine or faeces.

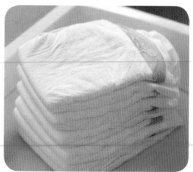

Bulk buy Until he is about four months old, you can expect to use up to 12 nappies each day. For this reason, it's worth buying nappies in bulk, to keep down the cost.

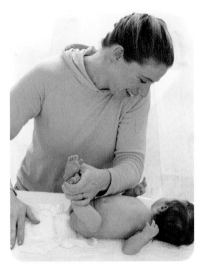

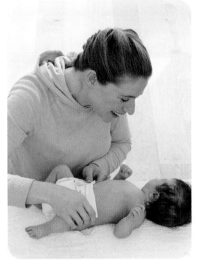

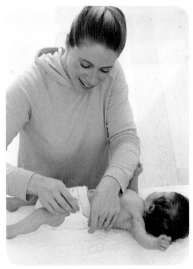

1 **With one hand,** hold your baby's legs together and lift his bottom. Place a clean nappy underneath, with the tabs just under his waist. For boy babies, make sure his penis is tucked down. Gently bring the nappy up between his legs.

2 **Make sure** the nappy fits comfortably between his legs, without too much bunching or gathering. Gently smooth the front, and then fasten the tabs securely. The nappy should feel snug but not too tight.

3 **Check that you can fit** a finger between the nappy and your baby's tummy, and that he's comfortable. Place your baby in a safe place where he cannot roll, and dispose of the used nappy. Always wash your hands carefully.

Nappy rash

Almost all babies suffer from nappy rash at some point, and it can be extremely uncomfortable. Nappy rash is caused by contact with urine or faeces, which cause the skin to produce less of its own protective oil and therefore provide a less effective barrier to further irritation.

Change frequently To avoid nappy rash it is important to change your baby often. You should also let him have some periods without a nappy at all, to allow air to circulate around his skin. Use fragrance-free wipes or fresh water when you clean his bottom.

Avoid chemicals Disposable nappies tend to be a little better at keeping urine away from the skin, so may be a short-term solution if you are using reusables. If you prefer reusable nappies, put them through an extra rinse cycle to make sure that there are no traces of detergent, and use a fragrance-free fabric softener.

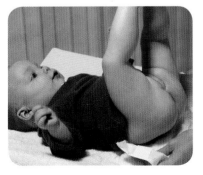

Sore bottom If your baby has nappy rash, his bottom will look red and sore, perhaps with little "pimples". If unchecked, the rash can spread up his front and across his buttocks.

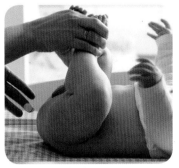

Barrier cream Although not essential at every change, zinc oxide cream provides a barrier between the contents of your baby's nappy and his skin.

Reusable nappies

With the environment in mind, and the development of easy-to-wash, practical, and easy-fastening varieties, many parents are choosing reusable nappies over disposables, and finding it a very viable option.

What to expect in your baby's nappy

In the days after her birth, your baby will pass "meconium", a thick, dark-green or black substance. This is perfectly normal.

★ **Breastfed babies** have frequent, often liquid bowel movements, that are yellow or yellowish green; they can contain little lumps, like milk curds.

★ **Formula-fed babies** normally have fewer bowel movements, which tend to be thicker and darker in colour.

★ **Hard, dry bowel movements** may be a sign of constipation or inadequate fluid intake. Speak to your midwife or GP.

★ **Any blood or mucus** in your baby's stool should be reported to your doctor.

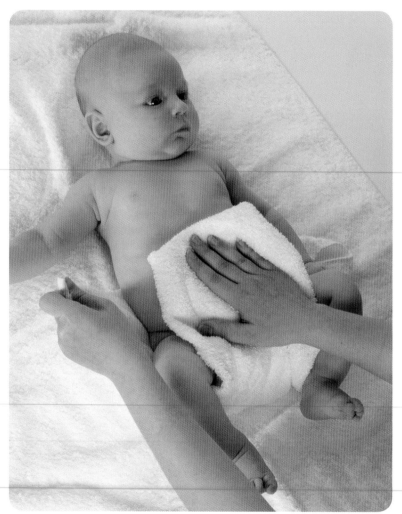

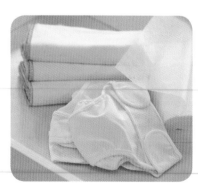

A good fit Reusable nappies are available in a variety of sizes, according to your baby's weight and age. If your nappies do not have a waterproof cover on the outside, you will need to buy waterproof pants.

Secure fastenings The days of sharp pins have long passed. There is now a variety of fastenings, including plastic nappy clips or "clamps" that are secured with a slide. Pre-folds come in a rectangular shape and are held in place by waterproof pants. Better still are shaped nappies fastened with Velcro or poppers, or covered by an outer wrap.

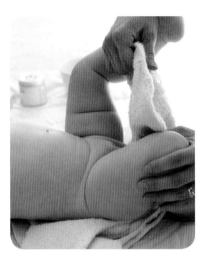

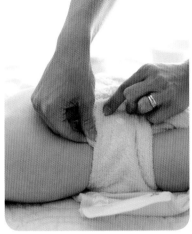

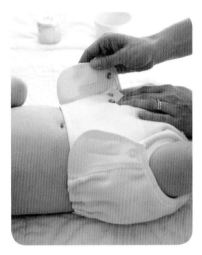

1 **Remove the soiled nappy,** and clean your baby's bottom. Spread a fresh nappy on a wrap, with a nappy liner on top. Although these can seem an unnecessary purchase, liners make it much easier to remove bowel movements, and help to keep moisture away from your baby's skin. Slide the nappy under her and spread a little barrier cream on her bottom.

2 **Fasten the nappy,** pinching the fabric between her legs to avoid bunching. The nappy should be securely fastened against your baby's tummy, but not too tight. You should be able to fit a finger between the top of the nappy and her tummy. Chat to your baby as you change her; she'll soon begin to associate nappy changing with fun.

3 **Secure the wrap** over the nappy, making sure that it is firmly fastened. Run your fingers around the legs to check that it completely covers the nappy, or you can expect some leakage. You can now dress your baby as usual. In most cases, you'll need to change your baby approximately every two hours, and always after she has had a poo.

Your baby's umbilical cord

Between five and 15 days after your baby's birth, the stump of your baby's umbilical cord will dry, blacken, and drop off. Underneath will be a small wound or sore that will heal over the next few days. It is completely normal for this area to look a little messy while it heals.

Keep it clean It is important to keep your baby's cord stump clean. Look for "bikini" nappies, which fasten below the umbilical area. These prevent irritation, and limit the possibility of faeces coming into contact with the stump. If you can't find this type, turn down the top of the nappy you are using, to leave the stump open to the air.

Look carefully You can expect a yellowish or even greenish discharge around the base of your baby's umbilical stump; but if the skin there becomes red or inflamed, or there is a smelly discharge, see your GP to rule out an infection.

Simple treatment Your baby's cord stump will be clamped with a plastic clip after she is born, and then checked in the hospital and during your home visits. It's no longer suggested that alcohol or antiseptic ointments, talc, or liquids be used on your baby's umbilical stump. Instead, plain, warm water will do the trick – with a little baby wash if the area becomes dirty. Always wash your hands carefully before cleaning around the cord. Use a thin, boil-washed flannel or cotton wool buds rather than balls, as little bits of loose fluff or threads from those can become caught around the stump, leading to irritation and infection.

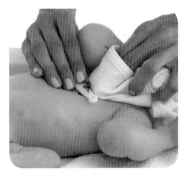

The stump Always wash your hands carefully before cleaning your baby's umbilical stump, and cleanse it gently.

Keeping your baby clean

A full bath isn't necessary every day, although it can be a lovely part of a relaxing bedtime routine. When your baby simply needs a gentle clean, you can "top and tail" him instead, sending him off to bed smelling fresh and clean.

Bathtime safety

★ **Never leave your baby** unattended in the bath – or near any source of water – even for a moment.

★ **Check the temperature** of the water carefully. The bath should be at the right temperature before you bathe him, and not topped up when he's in it.

★ **Consider using a slip mat** if you are bathing him in a full-sized bath. He'll be easier to hold and manage if he is in one position.

★ **If you choose to use** a baby bath, be sure that it is on a firm surface. Waist-height is ideal, to avoid having to bend and lift. If you do place it on the floor, make sure you hold your baby carefully before lifting him from the bath.

★ **Always keep** your baby's head supported in the bath.

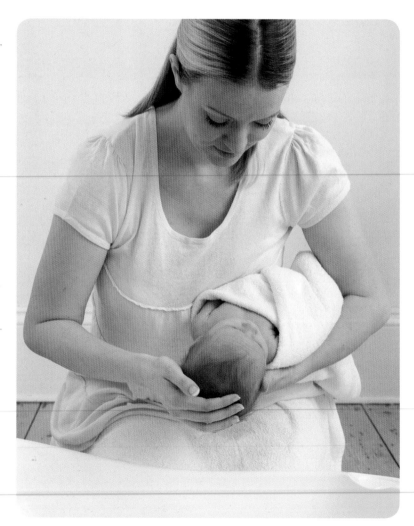

TOP TIP

If in doubt about the temperature of your baby's bath, use a bath thermometer. It should be 35–38°C/95–100°F. The lower end of the scale is best for a new baby.

1 **Check that the water** is not too hot. If you wish, you can add a few drops of baby bath to the water, which will help to remove dirt. Next, undress your baby and wrap him in a clean towel. Cradling him on one arm, lean him across the bath and wash his scalp with a wet, lightly soaped flannel. Rinse the flannel out and squeeze over his head.

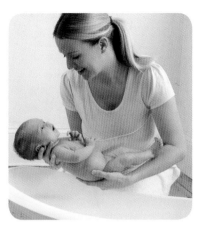

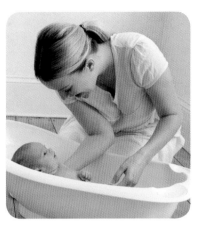

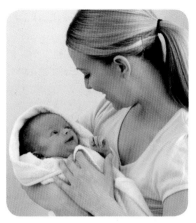

2 **Holding him securely,** lower your baby into the bath feet first, using one hand to support his neck and head. Use a thin flannel to clean him carefully, especially around any creases.

3 **Encourage him to have fun.** Splash the water a little, and sing and chat to him. It can be daunting to bathe a newborn, so try to stay upbeat or he may sense your anxiety.

4 **Wrap your baby** in a warm, dry towel immediately after bathing and hold him close. Hooded towels are great, as they prevent the loss of heat from his head and dry his hair at the same time.

Topping and tailing

To "top-and-tail" your baby, fill a sink or a bowl of warm water and add a few drops of baby bath. Then wash your baby in a place where he is most comfortable and away from any draughts. Make sure that you use different flannels for his face, body, and bottom, and always boil-wash them.

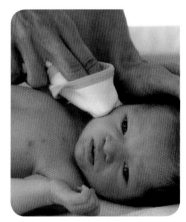

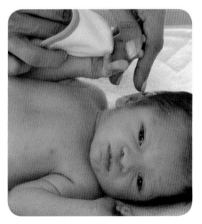

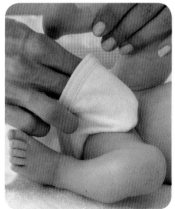

1 **Lay him on a firm surface** and, using a flannel, gently wash his face, behind his ears, and in the folds of his neck. A build-up of milk in these areas can cause irritation.

2 **Gently wash under** his arms, between his fingers, which can become surprisingly mucky, and across his tummy, but take great care with his umbilical stump (see p.159).

3 **Wash his genital area** gently, cleaning all the little creases and folds. Carefully turn him over, supporting his head as you do so, and wash his back, bottom, and legs.

Settling your baby down to sleep

Sleep can be elusive in the early days, but try to settle your baby while she is still awake, reassuring her until she feels secure enough to drift off. That way, she'll soon learn how to go to sleep herself, even if she wakes up in the night.

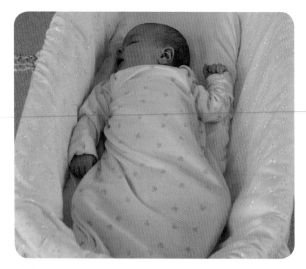

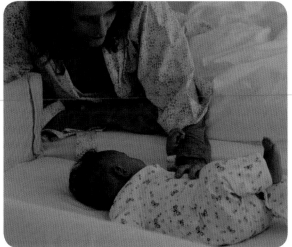

Secure space Many small babies feel more secure in a Moses basket or cradle. Avoid the temptation to overdress her. In warm weather, she may be comfortable in just a nappy with a blanket. Check her regularly, and add more layers if she seems cool.

Co-sleeper You may wish to purchase a "co-sleeper" cot that fastens onto your bed, making night-time breastfeeds easier. Your baby will enjoy having you close, but try not to pick her up every time she murmurs; she will usually go back to sleep on her own.

SIDS – Sudden Infant Death Syndrome

SIDS or "cot death" is the unexplained death of a baby. It occurs most frequently under the age of four months but can happen up to the age of four.

Although the cause is still unknown, extensive research has identified risk factors and some measures that can be undertaken to prevent it.

★ Keep your baby with you at all times until she is six months old.
★ Always put her down to sleep on her back, with her feet at the foot of her cot.
★ Keep her room temperature at around 18°C/64°F, and use layers of sheets and cellular blankets to avoid overheating.
★ Don't smoke during pregnancy and never let anyone smoke in the same room as your baby.
★ If your baby has a fever, she should be kept cool and seen by her doctor.
★ Don't share a bed with your baby if she is premature or you have been drinking alcohol or taking medication.

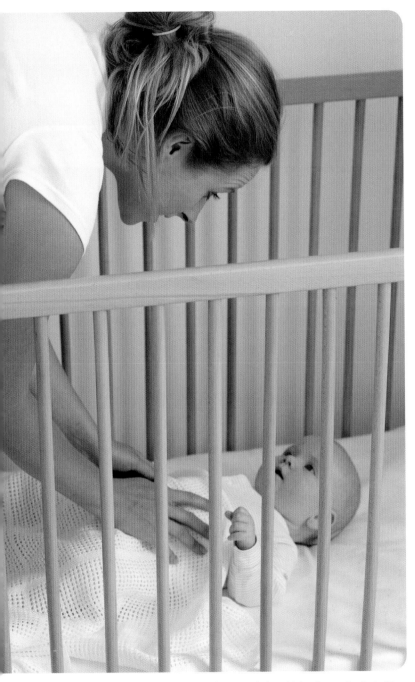

"Feet to foot" It is very important that you place your baby with her feet at the foot of her cot: "feet to foot". This not only helps to prevent cot death (see opposite), but can help to keep her blankets in place, as she can't wriggle down and under or away from them.

Helping your baby to sleep

★ Providing a comfort object, such as a favourite blanket or cuddly toy can help to reassure your baby. Many babies want to feel something familiar when they go to sleep or wake in the dark. A comfort object will also help your baby to settle when she isn't in her own cot.

★ Keep things quiet and low key in the run-up to bedtime. When she wakes in the night, feed and change her without engaging in any chat or play. She'll soon get the message that there is no fun to be had at night.

★ Settle her down for naps at regular intervals. Sometimes babies become over-tired and find it difficult to settle.

★ If she falls asleep feeding, gently wake her and make sure she is properly winded before being placed in her cot, otherwise she will be alarmed to find you gone when she wakes.

★ Try to avoid picking her up the moment she makes a noise. In many cases, she'll settle on her own.

★ A little complaining when she is left on her own is to be expected. Lay her down, and reassure her. If she cries, come back into the room and stroke her face or tummy until she feels happier, then leave the room again.

KEY FACT
Newborns should not be left to cry, no matter how many experts advocate "controlled crying". Crying is the only way for her to tell you that something is wrong.

Soothing and comforting your baby

Until you learn to understand and identify the cause of your baby's fussing, crying, and poor sleep, you may find some aspects of parenthood exhausting. The good news is that there are plenty of tried-and-tested techniques to help.

Soothing a crying baby

★ Many babies respond to being held and rocked, although you may find, frustratingly, that something that worked one day may not work the next.

★ Rhythmical sounds soothe many babies, such as low music, or even the sound of the vacuum cleaner.

★ If your baby is eased off to sleep by rocking, bring his pram or pushchair inside, and settle yourself in a position where you can comfortably rock him with a free hand or foot.

★ Some babies may feel more comfortable when "wrapped" in a blanket (see opposite).

★ Other babies may feel constrained by blankets and covers, and prefer a light blanket or a baby sleeping bag.

★ Some babies need to suck to get to sleep or to settle, which is why they feed almost constantly when they are upset. If he's not hungry, he may find some comfort from a dummy.

★ You may find that if you set up a routine that makes him feel secure (see p.148), he will calm down and feel more comfortable during the day.

★ If crying begins after feeding, after switching from breastmilk to formula, or after a change in formula, talk to your midwife or health visitor. There may be problems with the formula he is taking.

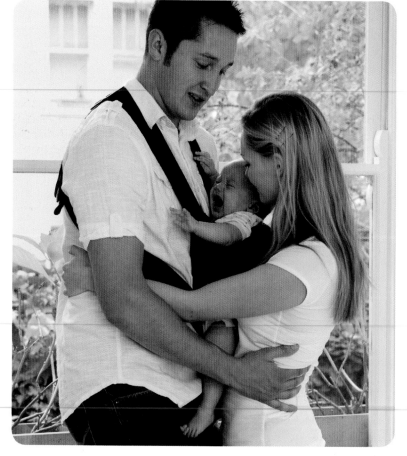

Keep him close Carrying your baby in a sling can help to soothe him, particularly if you aren't sure why he is distressed. Many babies like to have their heads near your chest, in order to hear your heartbeat. If he's been winded, his tummy is full, and he has a clean nappy, he may simply be over-tired, and respond best to some gentle rocking or walking.

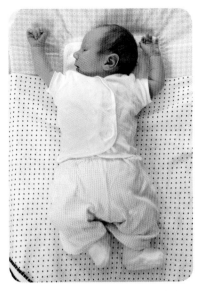

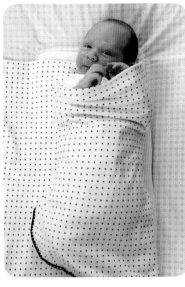

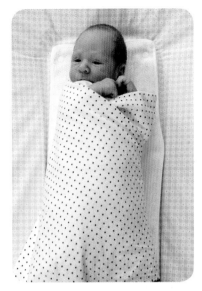

1 **Wrapping your baby** may help him to sleep more soundly if he tends to jerk himself awake. To wrap him, place him in the centre of a large blanket, with his arms and head above the top.

2 **Bring across the right-hand** side of the blanket, tucking it snugly, but not too tightly, underneath his body. It's important that his hands and forearms remain free of the blanket.

3 **Next, wrap the left-hand** side of the blanket around him, and tuck the edges beneath him. He should feel secure, but still able to move a little. You can then place him down to sleep.

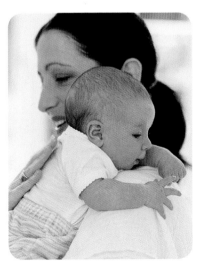

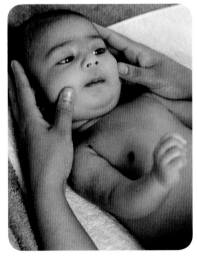

Trapped wind Swallowed air can be extremely uncomfortable for your baby, and it's worth winding him at the first sign of distress. Hold him upright and rub his back gently or pat him up and down his spine until you feel or hear the air released.

Massage A fractious, colicky baby may be soothed by a gentle massage (see pp.170–71). Massaging him before bed can help to relax him towards sleep, and if he tends to suffer from wind, it can also help to massage him before a feed.

Colic

Uncontrollable crying may be a sign of "colic" – generally thought to be a pattern of abdominal pain and crying that seems to occur at the same time each day.

Possible causes You can help by making sure that your baby is winded frequently during feeds, and, if you are breastfeeding, remove wind-producing foods such as cabbage, broccoli, and onions from your diet.

What to try Your GP may suggest anti-spasmodic drops to reduce discomfort. A warm bath can also help to ease symptoms. Colic can be distressing, but keep in mind that it almost always stops by three months.

Bonding with your baby

Bonding is not an event, but a process that grows and develops over months or even years. It encourages an intense, lasting attachment between parents and their babies, which involves love, affection, protection, and nourishment.

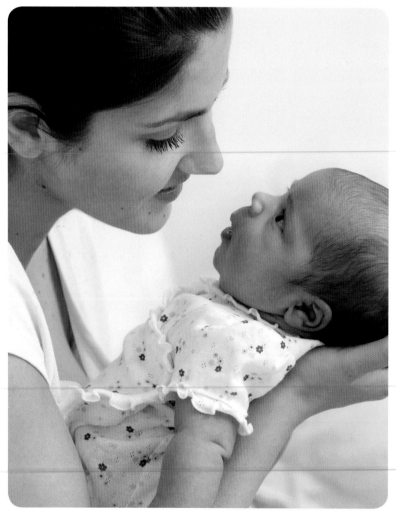

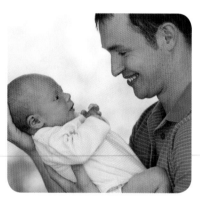

Male bonding Allow your partner space and time to develop his own routines and close relationship with his newborn. They'll both benefit from time alone together.

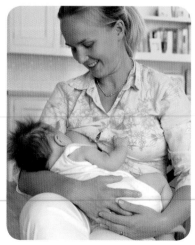

Physical closeness There is excellent research showing that breastfeeding can help to encourage the process of bonding and a strong mother-baby relationship.

The best investment Every moment that you spend with your baby will encourage the process of bonding, and deepen your attachment. Chat and sing to her, using plenty of eye contact. Watch how she responds to your facial gestures as she becomes older, and begins to mimic you. Respond to her little mews; you'll be holding your first conversation.

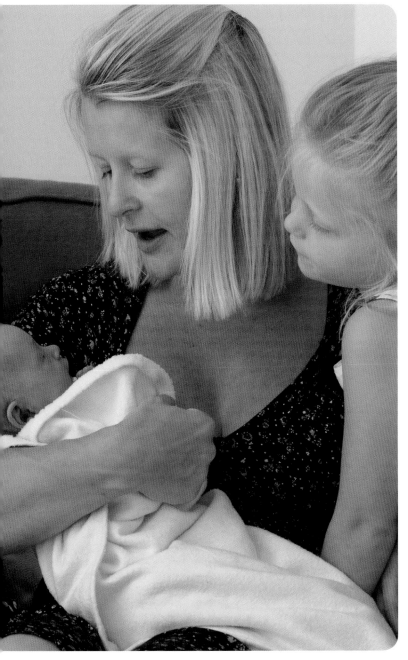

Making time for siblings

You can encourage a healthy relationship between your children – and help your other children feel loved and wanted – by making time for them all.

Older ones need you, too A new baby in the house can upset even the best-established routines, and leave your other children feeling out of sorts. It's important to remember that your newborn does have very defined needs, but as long as she's happy, clean, and well-fed, she'll be content. Her siblings need you most at this stage.

Find time Try to get a little help with your baby from time to time, so that you can settle down to read or play with your older children.

Be honest Above all, explain that a good proportion of mum and dad's attention will be taken up. If older children know what to expect, they will feel less disgruntled.

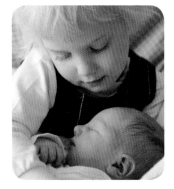

Be positive Encourage your toddler to be gentle with her new baby sister or brother and praise her efforts.

Include all your children Your other children will establish a healthy relationship with their new sibling over time, and you'll get things off to a flying start if you include them in your baby's care. They can pat your baby's tummy or feet when she is distressed, and even help to fetch and change nappies. Hold them all close together, so that they feel equally loved.

Getting to know your baby

The first weeks of your baby's life may pass in a blur, and you may wonder how you'll ever have time to regain some semblance of normal life; however, these long hours are well spent, as you get to know your baby and his unique personality.

Fun and games with your baby

Play is crucial for your baby's social, emotional, physical, and cognitive development. He will enjoy time spent playing with you as well as learning to explore the world around him – and a little of both will make sure that he is well-stimulated.

★ Even small babies will enjoy a baby gym, and from about two or three months your baby will be thrilled to find that he can make things happen with his erratic kicks. Choose one with highly contrasting colours and toys to bat at.

★ Tummy time is important for babies to develop strong back and neck muscles, and you can make it more fun by buying a textured baby mat.

★ Play music that your baby seems to enjoy, and use his reactions as a guide. Try a lively tune if he's happy or something soothing if he's fractious.

★ Sing or read silly rhymes and songs – this encourages an early appreciation and understanding of language.

★ When he's able to hold up his head, help him to stand up in your lap and bounce a little, which encourages gross motor skills.

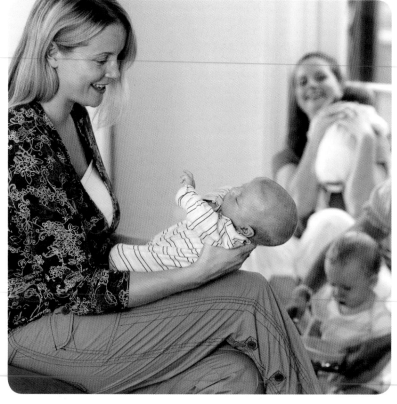

Get together Meeting other new mums provides a welcome opportunity to share your birth experience, and swap tips on coping with a newborn. These will be some of your baby's first "social" experiences, too, and it won't be long before he's playing alongside his new friends. Don't underestimate the importance of getting out and about. New motherhood can sometimes be lonely, and you'll feel more cheerful if you get a change of scene from time to time.

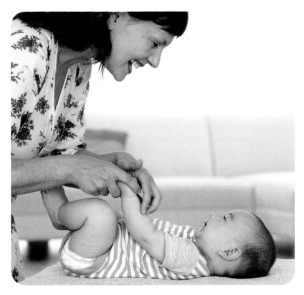

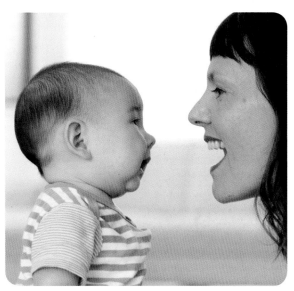

Enjoy some playtime Even very small babies will love to play, and you can gently tickle your baby, bicycle his little legs, and show him how his body works. Laugh, sing, and chat – he'll love to see your smiling face and hear your familiar voice. Every moment of time you spend together will help to cement your growing relationship.

Talk to him Exaggerate your facial movements, and he will soon begin to mimic you. He'll gaze at your face with wonder, and when that first magical smile appears somewhere around four or five weeks, you'll know that all your efforts have been worthwhile. Babies love to chat so talk and sing to him as often as you can.

Suitable toys

Your new baby can see only a short distance in front of his face, and he won't see everything in full colour for another few weeks; however, his sense of touch and hearing are very well developed, and he will enjoy experimenting with different sounds and textures.

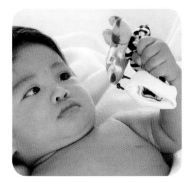

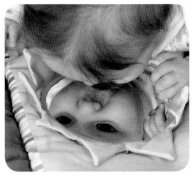

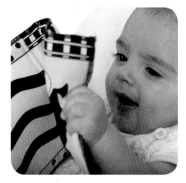

A rattle A soft rattle that makes a noise with just a little effort from your baby makes an ideal first toy.

A baby mirror It will be some time before your baby recognizes himself, but a mirror designed for young ones will entrance him.

Soft books It's never too early to introduce your baby to books. Choose soft ones with high-contrast patterns.

Baby massage

Massaging your baby is a wonderful way to relax your baby. It is also thought to encourage the process of bonding, and relieve discomfort, improve sleep, promote healthy weight gain, and even encourage cognitive development.

KEY FACT

One UK study found that massaging a baby can help to build better relationships between infants and mothers who have postnatal depression.

The importance of touch

The power of touch has been firmly established in conventional medicine, and it can encourage your baby's emotional and physical health on all levels.

You both benefit Massaging your baby is an excellent way of settling her, and of establishing a close physical relationship. She will feel loved and cared for, and you may find that you bond more easily. Touch is very therapeutic, and you will both benefit from loving contact.

Research studies The Touch Research Institute in the USA has found that premature babies massaged three times a day for as few as five days, consistently fare better than equally frail babies who don't get massages. Full-term infants and older babies also benefit from them. Parents who massage their babies report that it helps them to sleep better, relieves colic, and helps hyperactive children relax. New research shows that premature infants are more alert, sleep better, and gain weight more quickly when they are massaged regularly.

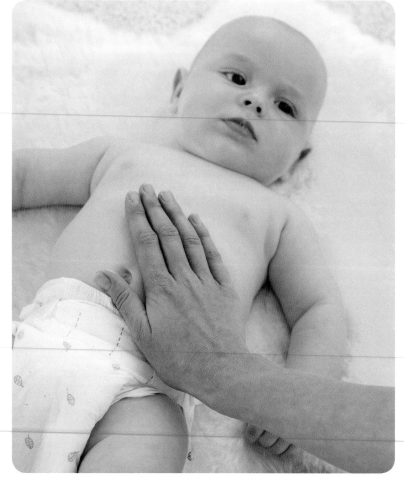

It's simple You don't need to learn any special strokes when you massage your baby; instead, simply use gentle rhythmic or stroking movements and let her reactions guide you. Choose a time when she is happy, and settle her on a safe surface, in a draught-free room.

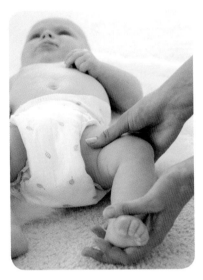

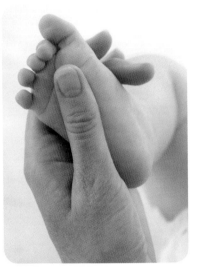

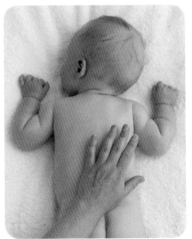

Using oils for baby massage

Oils can enhance massage but it's important that you choose those that are suitable for your baby.

Keep it simple Natural oils such as olive, grapeseed, or apricot kernel oil are perfect. Warm the oil in your hands first, and remember that your baby will be slippery afterwards. Rub off any excess with a clean, dry towel.

Check If you wish to use essential oils, consult a qualified aromatherapist who specializes in treating babies. Essential oils should only be used very sparingly (one drop to 60ml/2floz of carrier oil) and should not be used near your baby's mouth, eyes, or genitals.

Choose the right place and time If your baby is small enough, you can massage her on your lap. Alternatively, spread a towel on the floor. If your baby objects, wait until she is feeling calmer. Try massaging before a feed, or as part of the bedtime routine.

Have fun Make sure your baby is comfortable, and massage her gently from the top of her head to the tip of her little toes. While the aim is undoubtedly to soothe and relax her, there's no reason why you can't play games, too.

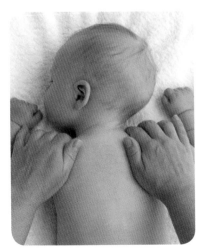

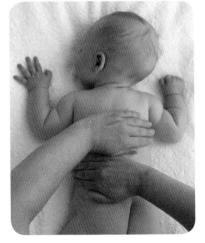

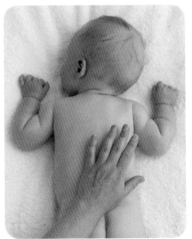

1 **If you are using oils** (see above), gently warm them in your hands first. Massage your baby from head to toe, placing her first on her back and then on her tummy. Stroke your baby's back – up and down, and in long, sweeping motions from her shoulders to her feet.

2 **Now, using a combination** of firm and gentle strokes, move your hands in both clockwise and anti-clockwise circles up and down your baby's body. As you massage with one hand, always keep the other resting gently on your baby's back to reassure her.

3 **With the palm** of your hand, gently press into the muscles of your baby's lower back. This is especially useful if she suffers from bouts of colic or frequent wind, as it relaxes the muscles of the lower digestive system. Singing and talking to her will enhance the experience.

Your first outing

It won't be long before you'll feel ready to take your baby a little further afield. Although it can be daunting to negotiate taking out a baby and his essential belongings on the first few occasions, you'll soon step into your stride.

Your baby's changing bag

Your baby's changing bag will become your "survival bag" when you are out and about, so it's important to keep it well organized. Consider including:

★ 3–5 clean nappies; if you are using reusables, make sure you have plastic pants and liners, too.

★ 2 plastic bags: for wet clothes and dirty or wet nappies.

★ Wipes and a flannel, for emergency all-over washes.

★ A small tub or tube of nappy or barrier cream.

★ 1–2 changes of clothes.

★ 1–2 boxes or tins of ready-prepared formula, if you aren't breastfeeding.

★ 1–2 clean, sterilized bottles with lids, if you aren't breastfeeding.

★ Nipple cream.

★ 1–2 muslin squares.

TOP TIP

There is no specific age at which you can take your baby on an outing. As long as you are feeling up to it, some fresh air and gentle exercise will do you both good.

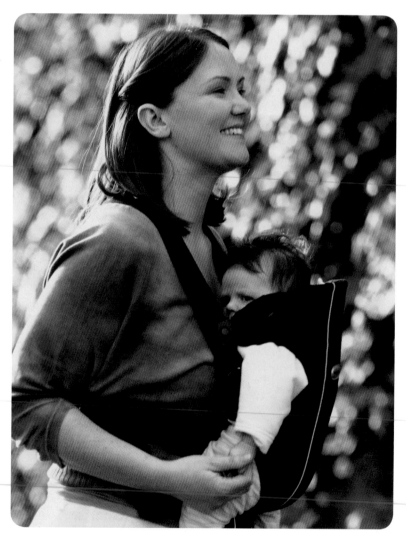

Hands-free A sling is the ideal way to carry your baby, leaving your hands free for shopping or a cup of tea with a friend. Your baby will love being close to your chest, and will probably settle down and sleep for most of your trips out of the house.

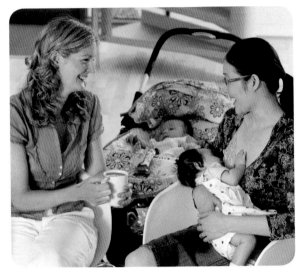

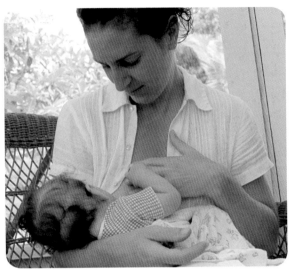

Make good use of the pushchair Your baby's pushchair will act as an impromptu seat and bed, allowing him to settle no matter where you are. Take the time to meet up with old and new friends; you'll find the change in your routine invaluable, and it can be reassuring to know that other mums share the same experiences.

Breastfeeding in public Some women find it embarrassing to breastfeed in public, even if it is the most natural act in the world. You can plot your trips according to the mother-and-baby rooms en route, or simply bring along a shawl or blanket to protect your modesty. Find a quiet spot and you'll find it much easier.

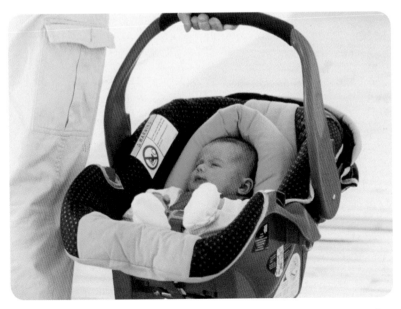

Easy transportation Your baby's car seat will undoubtedly become his favourite chair for the first few months of his life, and you can easily transport him in and out of the house or shops without disturbing him. For this reason, it's important to choose one with plenty of padding, a washable cover, and an easy-to-grip handle.

Spending time in his car seat

Portable car seats can mean that babies spend too much time sitting down.

Keep a check Baby car seats are now so portable that it is easy to lose track of how long your baby stays in the same position. Experts now advise that young babies should be transported in "stage one" carrycots or car seats that lie very flat. Medical research has shown that newborns who sit "scrunched up" in upright infant seats are potentially at risk of breathing problems. Furthermore, too much time spent in his car seat could limit your baby's opportunities for stimulation, which is necessary for him to develop sensory and motor skills.

173

Your support networks

In the past, many new mothers could depend on their extended families for help and support. Things are rather different these days, but that doesn't mean that you can't create your own networks to get what you need.

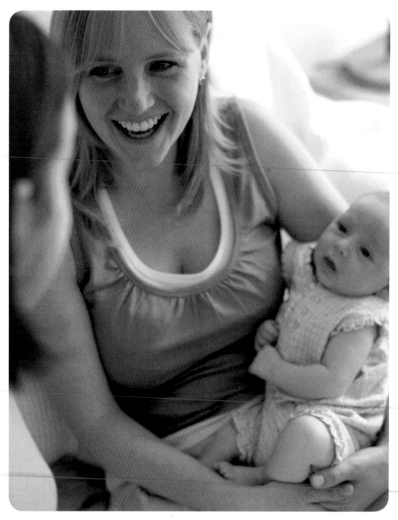

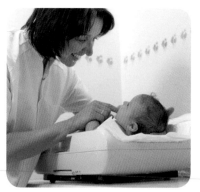

Regular checks Get into the habit of visiting your local baby clinic, to have your baby's weight and height plotted on her growth chart, and to discuss any worries.

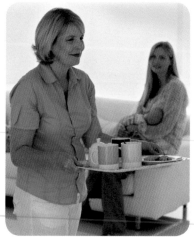

Accept help Your midwife will frequently see you at home after the birth of your baby, and at around 10–14 days a health visitor will visit. You can also go to a postnatal drop-in centre. These check-ups are to monitor your baby and to give you support and information. Make use of this professional expertise to help you find solutions to any concerns you may have.

Extended family Visits from family members can provide an opportunity to get a little rest, some help and advice, and another pair of hands to get the jobs done.

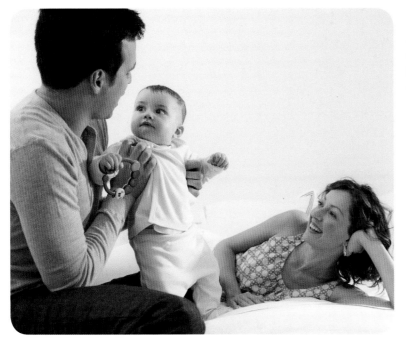

Support each other It's natural to feel tired and fractious with a new baby in the house, and you may find that you and your partner are snapping at each other. Remember that you are both in this together, and that empathizing with one another can help to make things much easier. Try not to be embarrassed about feeling overwhelmed, and support each other as much as you can. Time spent together as a new family can help to ease the pressure.

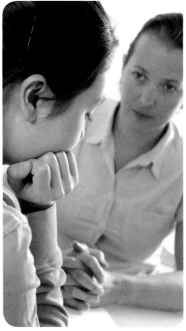

Get professional help If you are feeling depressed or unable to cope, see your doctor or health visitor as soon as possible. Postnatal depression can be easily treated, and your life can be made much happier.

Postnatal depression

Postnatal depression, which is different from the "baby blues" experienced by most women after the birth (see p.144), affects 10 to 15 per cent of all new mums. The symptoms differ between women, and it's normal to experience at least some of them after your baby's birth.

A new and different life The reality of life with a new baby – and your new responsibilities as a parent – can be quite overwhelming when you are probably feeling emotional and tired after the birth. However, if you suffer from one or more of the following symptoms regularly, and you aren't feeling any better after two weeks, it's time to get some help. Don't hesitate to talk to your doctor or midwife. Postnatal depression is common and treatable, and it's really important that you seek help before things get out of

hand. It's also worth noting that postnatal depression can strike well after your baby's birth, so if you just don't feel yourself and are struggling to cope, make sure you get the support you need. Symptoms may include:

★ Tearfulness
★ Anxiety
★ Guilt
★ Irritability
★ Confusion
★ Disturbed sleep
★ Excessive exhaustion

★ Difficulty in making decisions
★ Loss of self-esteem and a lack of confidence in your abilities as a mother
★ No enjoyment of motherhood
★ Fear of harming yourself or your baby
★ Hostility or a feeling of indifference to people you normally love
★ Difficulty in concentrating
★ Shame at being unable to be happy
★ Fear of judgment
★ Helplessness
★ Loss of libido
★ Loss of appetite

The transition to parenting

It can take some time to come to terms with your new roles, and to master the basics of babycare and parenting, so try not to expect perfection.

Positive parenting

★ Don't worry about being a perfect parent or following someone else's guidance. Work out your own ideas based on what it means to you to be a parent, and how you want to do it.

★ Talk through your fears and worries; there is a solution to everything if you remain calm and work as a team.

★ Make time for your relationship, and create regular opportunities to sort out issues as they arise, rather than bottling up resentment. Bringing up a baby is both rewarding and stressful, so you need to support one another.

★ Get organized. If you need help in the house, then don't hesitate to set it up. Make achievable lists for yourself, but don't fret if things don't get done. If both of you work to keep things ticking over, you'll have much more time for your relationship – and your new baby.

★ Take time for yourself. Parenting can be exhausting, and everyone needs a break to recharge their batteries and enjoy a little time on their own.

★ Eat healthy, whole foods and drink plenty of water. If your energy levels are even, you'll find it much easier to cope.

★ Take some regular exercise, which can help to reduce stress and keep you healthy and strong.

★ Trust your instincts.

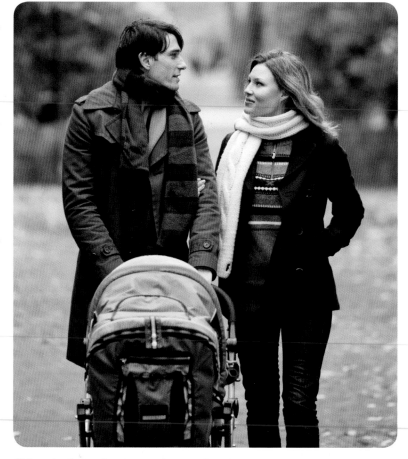

Walk and talk Spending time together away from the house and the daily chores can help you to gain perspective, and perhaps open up about the way you are feeling. There will be lots of important decisions to be made about your baby's care and your daily lives over the coming years, and it's good to get into the habit of having regular chats, to work out the best options.

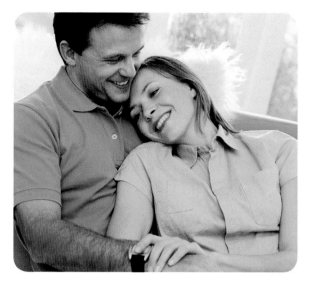

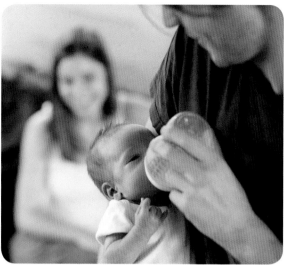

Cherish your partner, too Time alone, without your baby, is important to keep your relationship strong and healthy. The most effective, happiest parents are those that are able to maintain a good personal relationship as a couple, with plenty of opportunity to show affection, respect, appreciation, and, of course, love.

Enjoy sharing The responsibilities of parenting will give you both an opportunity to put your skills to the test, and you'll find that you each enjoy and shine at particular aspects of the job. The division of labour may never be entirely equal, but share it as much as you can. Your baby will love spending one-to-one time with both of you.

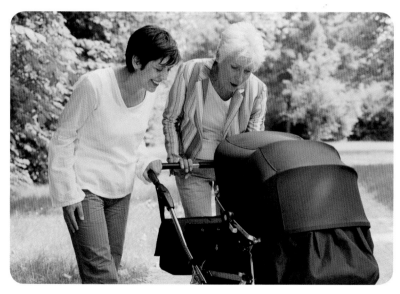

Special relationship Your baby's grandparents will enjoy the opportunity to help out whenever they can, and the relationship and bond that they develop with your little one will bring happiness to them and your baby. Although it can be difficult to accept what is sometimes dated advice, bear in mind that intentions are always good and your baby's grandparents may have a trick or two up their sleeves to get you through difficult times.

Including grandparents

Research shows that close, extended family relationships can have a positive impact on every area of your baby's life.

An important link Children with extended family contacts tend to be more literate, successful in their personal lives and happier. Your baby's grandparents will not just offer unconditional love, they will help to provide the optimum environment for him to learn everything from values, religious beliefs, table manners, respect, etiquette, social skills, responsibility, relationships, and even your family history. Don't underestimate how important this relationship will be for your child as he grows into a young man.

Adjusting to family life

Life as a family will be rewarding beyond your greatest expectations. Focus on the positives as you get to grips with looking after a newborn, and work on cementing the relationships that will remain strong for the rest of your lives.

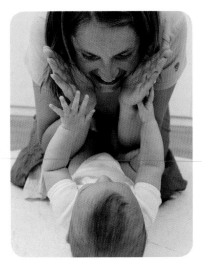

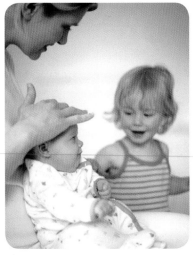

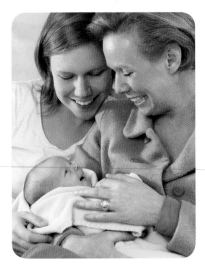

On your own Single parenthood is not easy, and you may sometimes find it hard to cope. However, the rewarding relationship you have with your baby will more than compensate.

Rivalry Your new arrival may provoke a little jealousy in your other children, so keep them involved and aware that they are important members of your family, too.

Extra help Your baby's extended family will offer love, warmth, and guidance as she grows – and may also be able to give you a welcome break from time to time.

Single parenting

The often negative press about the impact of single parenting on a child's life fails to take into consideration the wonderful bond that will be established between you and your baby. It's more difficult on your own, but that doesn't mean you won't give your baby the very best.

Accept help It is very important, to take time for yourself. An exhausted mother who gets little time on her own will undoubtedly struggle, so make use of any support networks that are available, and make sure that you get some rest. If you feel daunted making big decisions, talk to your friends and family – and ask your health visitor for advice. There are lots of organizations to provide you with support and guidance (see p.188). Take advantage of any tax breaks or credits, too – babies are expensive.

Keep dad involved If possible, encourage your baby's dad to have some role in his or her life. You may not be on great terms, but their relationship will be important in years to come and you may find that you can do a better job of co-parenting than being a couple.

Believe in yourself A single parent undoubtedly has a tougher job, but just as much love, as many good intentions, and plenty to offer a new baby. Your baby can and will thrive in your care.

Your new life When everything seems a bit overwhelming, look down at your amazing baby and take pride in your magnificent achievement. Things will settle down before you know it and you will revel in your new roles as parents.

Postnatal checks for mum

Between six and eight weeks after your baby's birth, you'll be given a full check-up by your GP to make sure that you are both physically and emotionally well.

TOP TIP

You can resume sexual relations with your partner as soon as it feels comfortable, but if you do experience pain or discomfort, see your doctor.

Your postnatal check

Your doctor will probably ask you the following questions:

★ How was your baby delivered?

★ Do you have any concerns or questions about your general health and wellbeing?

★ Is your perineum or Caesarean scar healing well?

★ Is your discharge normal, and have your periods resumed?

★ Are both your bladder and bowel functioning normally?

★ Are you breastfeeding?

★ How are you feeling about the birth experience?

★ How is your mood?

★ What is your diet like and are you taking any exercise?

★ How are you sleeping?

★ Have you considered which form of contraceptive you will now use?

★ Do you smoke?

★ Are you well supported at home?

★ Do you have any worries or concerns about your baby?

★ Is your baby content, healthy, and growing, as well as responsive?

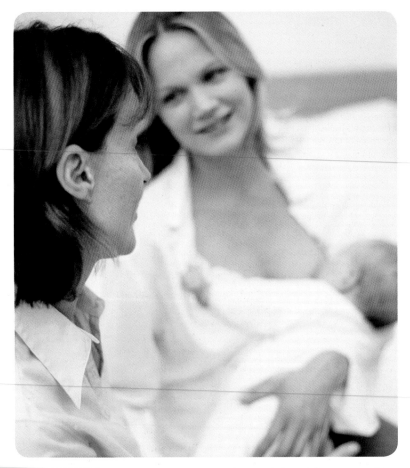

Be open Your doctor will ask about how you are feeding your baby and discuss any problems you may have. She'll ask how you are feeling – if you are finding things difficult, don't be afraid to admit it. While the "blues" are normal, postnatal depression (see p.175) poses a risk to both you and your baby, but your doctor can help, so take advantage of her concern.

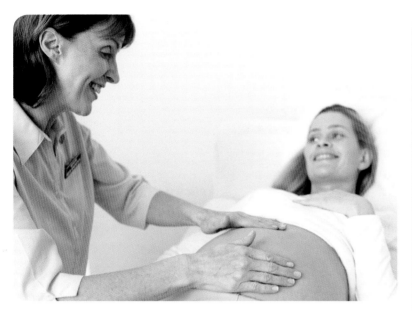

Physical examination Your doctor will check that everything has returned to normal after the birth. She'll palpate your uterus to be sure that it has contracted, and discuss any discharge or bleeding that may still be present. If you've had a Caesarean, she'll take a good look at your scar; if you've had stitches to your perineum, the site will be examined as well. An internal examination is not normally required.

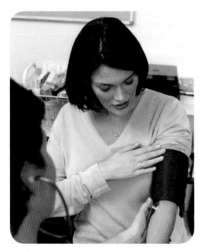

Tests Your blood pressure will be taken, and if you suffered from diabetes during pregnancy, your urine and blood will be checked. Women who had anaemia during pregnancy may also have a test to be sure that their iron levels have returned to normal.

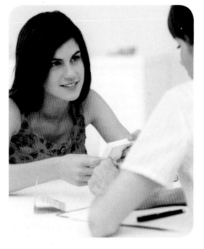

Birth control Contraception will be discussed and your doctor will help you choose the method that suits you best. Although breastfeeding can help to prevent you from becoming pregnant during this period, it is by no means infallible.

Exercising after the birth

Soon after birth you can start some pelvic floor exercises (see pp.30–31) and perhaps some tummy exercises, but make sure that you only do what feels comfortable.

Take care You may find exercise tricky if you have had a Caesarean, so go at your own pace and stop if you feel uncomfortable.

Begin gently Try some simple stretching when your baby is sleeping – or in his chair beside you. He'll be intrigued by your activities, and enjoy the company. Stretch only to the point where you are comfortable; the muscles and ligaments in your body will have softened and stretched during pregnancy and may take some time to return to normal. Swimming is a wonderfully relaxing aerobic exercise, and you can safely begin when your bleeding has stopped.

Feel good Exercise can lift your mood dramatically, encouraging the release of happy hormones known as endorphins. It's also a great way to release stress.

Maintain energy levels Try not to worry too much about losing weight. If you are breastfeeding, you'll need to eat well to ensure your milk supply and the nutrient content of your milk, and you'll need plenty of energy to keep up with the demands of parenthood. If you stick to a diet of healthy, fresh, whole food and give the biscuit tin a miss, the weight will begin to fall off naturally. Combined with some regular exercise, you'll soon regain your pre-pregnancy shape.

Postnatal checks for your baby

Around the same time that you have your own postnatal check, your baby will be given a full examination to make sure that she is thriving.

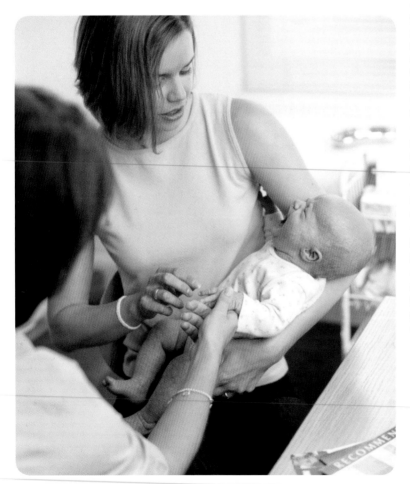

Reassure her Your baby may not relish the idea of having her clothes removed for a full examination, but try to stay calm. Soothe her, sing to her, and bring along a comfort item that may reassure her. You may need to stop and give her a short feed to relax her enough to continue. Try not to worry. All doctors are aware that babies do not always cooperate.

Your baby's check:

All of the findings will be recorded in your baby's health record book.

★ **Your baby will be checked** from head to toe. Her eyes will be examined using an ophthalmoscope. Her mouth, ears, neck, hands, and feet will be checked, and her head control and limb tone tested. Her chest, abdomen, spine and her anus will also be examined. A boy will be examined to check that his testicles have descended.

★ **Her hearing will be tested.** Your doctor will ask you whether she is startled when she hears a loud noise, and starting to make cooing noises.

★ **You will be asked** about your baby's vision – does she fix your face with her eyes and follow you with them?

★ **Your baby's tummy** will be felt and her hips will be checked for signs of instability or dislocation.

★ **You'll be asked how well** she is sleeping and if she is sleeping on her back, which is now recommended to prevent SIDS (see p.162).

KEY FACT
If your baby is on roughly the same centile line that she was when she was born, there is no need for concern. Some children are just smaller and slighter than others.

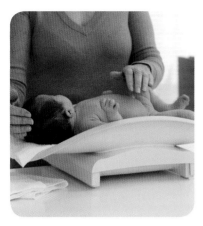

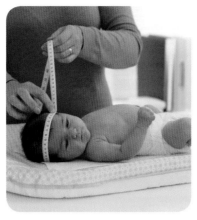

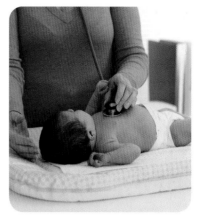

Weight Your baby will be weighed and her measurements recorded in her health record book. Your doctor will plot her weight on her growth chart, to check that she stays on roughly the same centile line as she was at birth. It's normal for babies to lose weight in the first week or so, but by the time she has her check, she should be back on target.

Growth Your baby's length and head circumference will be measured. Again, these figures will be plotted on her growth charts to check that she is growing as expected. Don't be surprised if she dips a little from time to time. This is completely normal, and will be recovered when she has her first major growth spurt.

Breathing and pulse Your GP will listen to your baby's heart. If she had a minor heart murmur at birth, your doctor will check to see if it has disappeared. If there are any problems, you will be referred to a specialist who can rule out any abnormalities. Your baby's breathing will also be checked to make sure that she isn't struggling.

Immunization

Routine immunization begins at about eight weeks of age, when your baby will receive the first of a series of vaccinations designed to prevent her from contracting the most serious childhood illnesses. While it can be upsetting to see your baby have these first jabs, she'll soon recover.

Go prepared Your baby may experience a little discomfort during the procedure, so it can help to bring along a comfort item or her dummy, and to talk to her throughout. Afterwards it is normal for your baby's temperature to elevate slightly, and for her to be a little more tired and grumpy than usual. If she experiences any other symptoms, such as a very high fever, vomiting, or a rash, call your doctor immediately. In most cases, a little paracetamol will ease her discomfort.

Keep a record It's a good idea to note down the date of each immunization (although this may vary between health authorities), and to record any symptoms or side-effects. You may need this information later, as your baby gets older.

Age	Vaccine
★ 2 months	5 in 1 (tetanus, diphtheria, pertussis (whooping cough), Hib (influenza type B), and polio) Pneumococcal infection
★ 3 months	5 in 1, Meningitis C
★ 4 months	5 in 1, Meningitis C, Pneumococcal infection
★ 12 months	Hib, Meningitis C
★ 13 months	MMR (measles, mumps, and rubella), Pneumococcal infection

What next?

Your baby's first few months of life will literally fly by and he will grow and develop at an astonishing rate. Your helpless new baby will soon have a mind of his own, and a personality to match, so enjoy him.

Your baby's development

By three months, your baby may:

★ Grasp items reflexively.

★ Lift his head.

★ Coordinate his sucking, swallowing, and breathing.

★ Smile socially.

★ Stop crying when he is picked up.

★ Use a different cry when he is tired, hungry, or in pain.

★ Coo when he is spoken to.

★ Visually recognize his parents.

★ Visually track moving objects or faces from 20–25cm (8–10in) away.

★ Look in the direction of sounds.

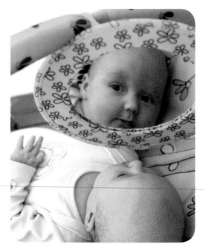

Play is vital Everything that your baby does will enhance his development. Don't underestimate the importance of play; it's all part of learning about the world around him and developing his coordination skills.

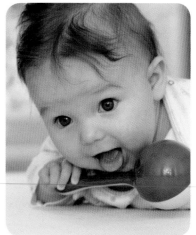

Head control By the end of his first month, your baby will be able to lift his head for short periods, and turn it from side to side, when he is on his tummy. By six months he'll have mastered this skill reliably.

Choosing a babysitter

On the first few occasions, it can be worrying to leave your baby alone with someone else; however, everyone needs a reliable babysitter from time to time, and taking steps to find one that is right for you and your baby will make you feel much more confident and happy about leaving him.

Someone you trust You may use a close friend or family member for the first few outings. Explain your baby's routine, the things that may settle him, and how often you expect him to be fed and changed.

Check carefully Always interview a babysitter before taking him or her on.

You'll also need to get and follow up references. Look for a babysitter with experience of new babies, and, ideally, a first-aid certificate. Babysitters must be at least 16 years of age; young ones can be particularly good if they've got younger siblings of their own, but make sure they can confidently cope with your baby.

Introduce them Make sure that you introduce your baby to his sitter in advance of any evenings or days out. He may be asleep for most of your outing, but if he wakes, he'll need to see a familiar face. Always leave your mobile number and your doctor's contact details by the telephone.

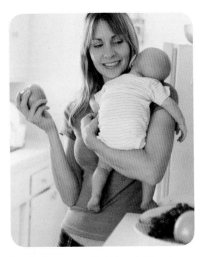

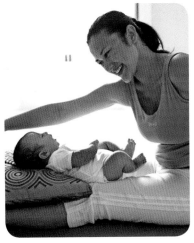

Look after yourself Although life gets easier as the weeks go by, motherhood is demanding and you'll need to take care of yourself. Make sure you have a healthy diet, with plenty of fresh, whole foods. Snacks will keep you going, but choose healthy ones to keep your blood-sugar levels steady.

Get back into shape If this is a priority for you, there's no reason why you can't involve your baby, too. He'll love watching your actions, and will find the repetition entertaining. Even a little stretching during his playtime can help you to regain your fitness and feel more energetic.

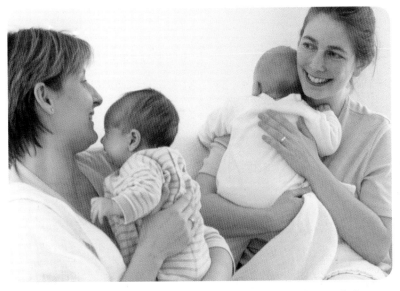

A new perspective One of the most wonderful aspects of parenthood is introducing your baby to a whole new set of experiences. Everything you do with him will be interesting and entertaining, and you may find that you also view the world around you with new eyes. There are plenty of fun activities that are suitable for little ones, and from about six or eight weeks you can take your baby for his first swim.

Maintaining your pre-baby social life

It may seem impossible to fit in all the activities you once did, but it's worth making an effort. A little time away helps you to relax properly and gain some perspective.

Make the effort You may tear out your hair trying to get ready in time, but it's well worth making the effort to go out and socialize. Not only will it offer you a magnificent opportunity to show off pictures of your new baby, but a little time away helps you to recharge your batteries.

New interests Although the activities you choose may be slightly different to those you pursued before you became pregnant, a chat with your friends, a meal out, or a trip to the cinema can offer welcome respite from the demands of parenthood. There is evidence that this type of activity can help to prevent postnatal depression, too.

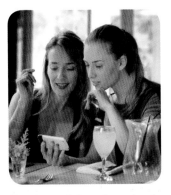

Keep in touch Some time out and about with friends will lift your spirits and give you a well-deserved break.

Enjoying your new baby

Your baby will change enormously over the coming months, so it is incredibly important that you take time simply to appreciate and enjoy her company.

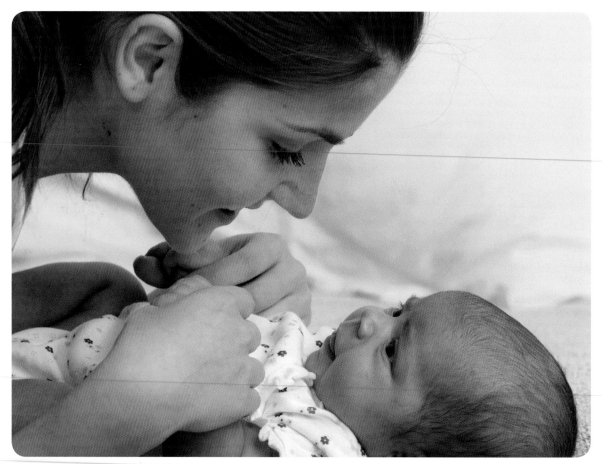

Mutual adoration Babies are easily amused and will show great pleasure at the simplest things. The sound of your voice, the familiar sight of your face close to hers, a warm cuddle, and a playful game of peek-a-boo will entertain her almost endlessly. What's more, she'll become increasingly confident and secure in the knowledge that you love her unconditionally and have all the time in the world for her. Even the most frustrated, irritable mum can't help but melt in the presence of an adoring little face looking up at her!

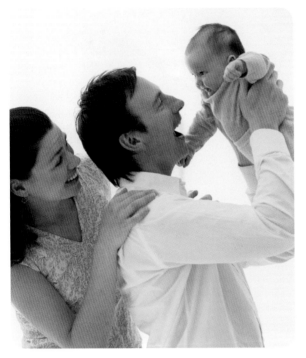

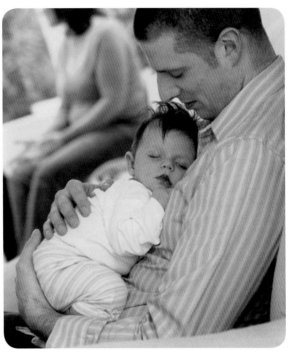

Time well spent Although it can be tempting to get on with chores when your partner looks after your baby, it is important to spend time as a family. Not only will it help to cement your relationship, but your baby will become more secure in a close family unit.

Magic moments The time you spend alone with your baby will provide a magical opportunity to bond. Your unconditional love will shine through in everything you do, so never worry about doing things "right". Instead, revel in the moments you have together.

Trusting your instincts

Parenthood can leave you reeling between infatuation, delight, complete bewilderment, and exhaustion. Try to remember that there is no "right" way to do things, and that your instincts are probably correct. So try to relax from time to time and give yourself a break.

You can do it No parent is perfect and there is no one way to raise a healthy, happy baby. We increasingly rely on handbooks that can be incredibly prescriptive, and undermine our confidence. The best advice however, is to trust your instincts and use the helpful tips offered as a basis for your very own, individual form of babycare. Rest assured that your love for your baby is the most important thing you can offer her, and as long as she is safe, clean, nourished, and gently stimulated, she'll thrive.

You know your baby best There will be times when you are unsure of how to deal with problems. Your health visitor, doctor, and even parents and friends can probably give you lots of solutions that may not have been immediately evident, and you can choose the best approach based on your circumstances, but trust in your instincts too. This is particularly relevant when your baby is ill. Anything out of the ordinary, such as a high fever, unusual bowel movements, extreme floppiness or sleepiness, vomiting,

diarrhoea, or strange rashes should of course, be seen by your doctor; however, you may also have a sense that something is not right. Go with your feelings, and trust yourself.

Enjoy it Those early days will soon pass, and you will begin not just to recognize what your baby's different cries mean, but to know exactly how to comfort her. As your life slips into a gentle routine, you'll be able to relax and enjoy your role as parents. This is where the real fun begins!

Useful resources

PREGNANCY

Action on Pre-eclampsia
www.apec.org.uk
020 8427 4217

Antenatal Results and Choices
www.arc-uk.org
020 7631 0285

The British Wheel of Yoga
For finding a pregnancy yoga class
www.bwy.org.uk
01529 306851

Eating for Pregnancy
www.eatingforpregnancy.co.uk

The Ectopic Pregnancy Trust
www.ectopic.org.uk
020 7733 2653

Pilates Foundation
For Pilates classes for pregnancy
www.pilatesfoundation.com
020 7033 0078

QUIT
Provides practical help, advice and
support by trained counsellors to
smokers who want to stop
www.quit.org.uk
0800 00 22 00

**Royal College of Obstetricians
and Gynaecologists**
www.rcog.org.uk
020 7772 6200

LABOUR AND BIRTH

Active Birth Centre
www.activebirthcentre.com
020 7281 6760

BirthChoiceUK
Information on choosing where to
have your baby and whom you
choose to look after you in labour
www.birthchoiceuk.com

Doula UK
www.doula.org.uk

Home Birth
www.homebirth.org.uk

Independent Midwives UK
www.independentmidwives.org.uk
0845 4600 105

Royal College of Midwives
www.rcm.org.uk
020 7312 3535

BABY

**Association of Breastfeeding
Mothers**
www.abm.me.uk
08444 122 949

Breastfeeding Network
www.breastfeedingnetwork.org.uk
0300 100 0210

**International Association of
Infant Massage (UK)**
www.iaim.org.uk
020 8989 9597

National Breastfeeding Helpline
www.breastfeeding.nhs.uk
0300 100 0212

La Leche League
www.laleche.org.uk
0845 456 1855

RIGHTS AND BENEFITS

**Advisory, Conciliation and
Arbitration Service**
www.acas.org.uk
08457 474 747

Citizens Advice
www.citizensadvice.org.uk

Child Benefit help
www.hmrc.gov.uk
0845 302 1444

Directgov Tax Credits help
www.direct.gov.uk
0845 300 3900

**Department for Work and
Pensions**
www.dwp.gov.uk

**Equality and Human Rights
Commission**
www.equalityhumanrights.com
0845 604 6610

Inland Revenue Tax Credit help
www.taxcredits.inlandrevenue.gov.uk
0845 300 3900

Maternity Action
www.maternityaction.org.uk
020 7253 2288

Working Families
www.workingfamilies.org.uk
0800 013 0313

SUPPORT GROUPS

Association for Post-Natal Illness
www.apni.org
020 7386 0868

Bliss
Support for families of premature
and special care babies
www.bliss.org.uk
0500 618 140

Down's Syndrome Association
www.downs-syndrome.org.uk
0845 230 0372

Miscarriage Association
www.miscarriageassociation.org.uk
01924 200 799

Postnatal Illness
www.pni.org.uk

**Stillbirth and Neonatal Death
Charity**
www.uk-sands.org
020 7436 5881

GENERAL

Fatherhood Institute
www.fatherhoodinstitute.org
0845 634 1328

Family Planning Association
www.fpa.org.uk

Gingerbread
Advice and information for
one-parentfamilies
www.gingerbread.org.uk
0808 802 0925

Home Start
Support for families in local
communities
0800 0686 368
www.home-start.org.uk

National Childbirth Trust
www.nct.org.uk
0300 330 0772

Parentline Plus
www.parentlineplus.org.uk
0808 800 2222

**Twins and Multiple Birth
Association**
www.tamba.org.uk
0800 138 0509

Tommy's, the baby charity
Research on miscarriage, premature
birth and stillbirth
www.tommys.org
020 7398 3483

Twinsclub
www.twinsclub.co.uk

Index

Acknowledgments

AUTHOR'S ACKNOWLEDGMENTS:

I would like to thank my family and friends who have supported me during the writing of this book. Thank you, also, to my midwifery and obstetrics colleagues who have kept me updated with the latest information to guide expectant parents through pregnancy, birth and the transition to parenthood.

A very special thank you to Karen Sullivan, the consultant editor, for her help, and everyone at DK who made the book possible, especially Helen Murray, Claire Tennant-Scull, Sara Kimmins, Carolyn Hewitson, Penny Warren, Glenda Fisher and Peggy Vance.

PUBLISHER'S ACKNOWLEDGMENTS:

DK would like to thank Angela Baynham for editorial assistance and proofreading, Kate Meeker for editorial assistance, Susan Bosanko for the index; Jo Godfrey-Wood for assistance at photo shoots; Victoria Barnes and Roisin Donaghy for hair and make-up; Carly Churchill, the photographer's assistant, and our models: Danielle Valliere and Tom and Dylan Baird; Emma Godden and Paul Bromage; Axl Habanananda; Alaina Powell; Jonica and Richard Thomas; Marcella Woods and Michael-Gabriel Fiori-Woods.

The publisher would like to thank the following for their kind permission to reproduce their photographs:

(Key: a-above; b-below/bottom; c-centre; l-left; r-right; t-top)

Alamy Images: Moose Azim / Bubbles Photolibrary 67tr; Dionne McGill 145br; Daniel Pangbourne / Bubbles Photolibrary 58r; Picture Partners 109tc; Chris Rout 46tl; **Babybond® www.babybond.com:** 55cr; **Corbis:** Rick Chapman 49t; **CJPG / Zefa 34; Eyetrigger Pty Ltd.** 82cra; Adam Gault / Science Photo Library 14bc; Brownie Harris 134; Michael A. Keller 21br; Beau Lark 175tl; Mika 36cra; Tetra Images 139br; Larry Williams 86-87; **Dreamstime.com:** Monkey Business Images 14cra; **Getty Images:** altrendo images 167br; Terry Anderson 146; Blend Images / Andersen Ross 69bl; Blend Images / Jose Luis Pelaez Inc. 16b, 54l, 58l; Blend Images / Jose Luis Pelaez, Inc. 105; Blend Images / Terry Vine 76c; Brand X Pictures / Steve Allen 64cra; Comstock Images / Thinkstock 93, 173tr; Cultura / Aurelie and Morgan David de Lossy 178r; Digital Vision / Rayes 21tr; Digital Vision / Trinette Reed 35tc; DK Stock / Christina Kennedy 14ca; George Doyle 11; First Light / Roderick Chen 135l; FoodPix / Anthony-Masterson 185tl; Adam Gault / SPL 95t; Nicole Hill 40cr; Ian Hooton / SPL 19tr; Iconica / Jamie Grill 36bc; Iconica / ML Harris 40bc; Image Source 21tl, 38ca; The Image Bank / Jonathan Storey 103br; The Image Bank / LWA 60ca; The Image Bank / MoMo Productions 29; The Image Bank / PictureGarden 185br; iStock Exclusive / Martin Carlsson 132l, 132r, 133l, 133r; Jose Luis Pelaez Inc 140-141; Nordic Photos / Michael Jonsson 33tr; OJO Images / Ashley Gill 177tr; OJO Images / Chris Ryan 92bc; OJO Images / Paul Bradbury 36ca; PhotoAlto / Eric Audras 181bc; PhotoAlto / John Dowland 46tc; Photodisc 89; Photodisc / Andersen Ross 131l; Photodisc / Blasius Erlinger 32; Photodisc / Jacqueline Veissid 37; Photodisc / Loungepark 46bc; Photodisc / Marcy Maloy 59, 62; Photographer's Choice / Nancy Brown 47; Photographer's Choice RF / Jacobs Stock Photography 12br; Photographer's Choice RF / Maria Spann 71bl; Photolibrary 109b; Photonica / Betsie Van Der Meer 12bc; Photonica / Gavin Kingcome Photography 38bc; PhotosIndia.com 57; Plattform 176; Riser / Frank Herholdt 119, 138; Riser / Hans Neleman 174cra; Riser / Jakob Helbig 12cra; Riser / Sam Royds 68; Sonntag 8-9; Stockbyte 38cla, 41; Stockbyte / Diane Macdonald 135r; Stone / Barbara Maurer 177b; Stone / Luca Trovato 127t; Taxi / Andreas Pollok 43br; Taxi / Bill Ling 13; Taxi / Caroline von Tuempling 15br; Taxi / Steen Larsen 21bl; Tetra Images 113bl; Workbook Stock / Stephen Chiang 121t; **Lennart Nilsson Image Bank:** Scanpix 50; **Life Issues Institute:** 52bl; **LOGIQlibrary:** 54cr; **Masterfile:** 38ca; **Mother & Baby Picture Library:** 33tl; Dave J. Anthony 21bc; Moose Azim 94bl, 114bl; Ian Hooton 15bl, 16cr, 17tl, 18, 19tc, 26ca, 33br, 35b, 56ca, 56cra, 66, 70, 88bl, 90bc, 90br, 94br, 101bl, 102, 104c, 108, 124, 174l, 178c, 181bl, 182, 185tc; Ruth Jenkinson 99r, 122, 125tl, 130; Eddie Lawrence 91tr, 129t, 142bl; Paul Mitchell 26cra, 88bc; James Thomson 99l; Frances Tout 121b; **Photolibrary:** Bananastock 118; BSIP Medical / Chassenet 46br; Digital Vision 1, 61; Graham Monro 128; Greg Newington 46bl; Vladimir Pcholkin 20; Radius Images 116; **PunchStock:** Blend Images 42; **Dept of Fetal Medicine, Royal Victoria Infirmary:** 55br; **Science Photo Library:** 56cb; AJ Photo 56crb, 126bl, 175tr; Anatomical Travelogue 51br; Samuel Ashfield 129b; B. Boissonnet 67tl; Neil Borden 55tc, 55tl; Neil Bromhall 52tl; Neil Bromhall / Genesis Films 51bl; BSIP, Laurent 95bl, 111bl, 125tr; CC Studio 157bc; Kevin Curtis 53; Tracy Dominey 127b; Dopamine 51tl; Edelmann 52br; Ian Hooton 10bl, 14br, 17tr, 98, 111tr, 180, 181t; Ruth Jenkinson / Midirs 91tl; Eddie Lawrence 126r; Dr. Najeeb Layyous 65; Living Art Enterprises, LLC 55bc, 55bl; Damien Lovegrove 40br; Cecilia Magill 10bc; Dr. P. Marazzi 38br; Doug Martin 64cla; Professor P. M. Motta Et Al 12ca; Lea Paterson 58c; Antonia Reeve 126cla; P. Saada / Eurelios 54cra; James Stevenson 52tr; Tek Image 123tr; Silvere Teutsch / Look At Sciences 117bl; John Thys / Reporters 101br; Zephyr 51cra; **Winchester and Eastleigh Healthcare NHS Trust:** 90ca

All other images © Dorling Kindersley
For further information see: www.dkimages.com